THE YOGA
OF POWER

Other Books by Julius Evola
from Inner Traditions International:

The Doctrine of Awakening
Eros and the Mysteries of Love
The Hermetic Tradition
The Mystery of the Grail
Revolt Against the Modern World

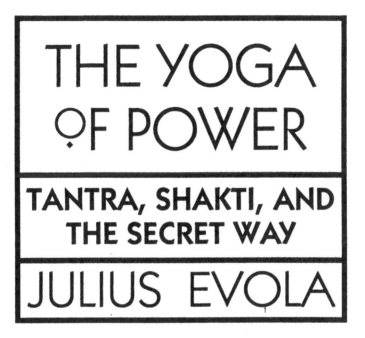

THE YOGA OF POWER

TANTRA, SHAKTI, AND THE SECRET WAY

JULIUS EVOLA

Translated by Guido Stucco

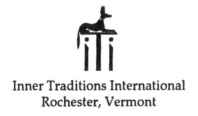

Inner Traditions International
Rochester, Vermont

Inner Traditions International
One Park Street
Rochester, Vermont 05767
www.InnerTraditions.com

First published in Italian under the title *Lo Yoga Della Potenza: Saggio sui Tantra*
by Edizioni Mediterranee, Rome, 1968

First U.S. edition 1992

Library of Congress Cataloging-in-Publication Data

Evola, Julius, 1898–1974.
    [Yoga della potenza. English]
    The yoga of power : tantra, shakti, and the secret way / Julius
Evola ; translated by Guido Stucco.
        p.   cm.
    Translation of : Lo yoga della potenza.
    Includes bibliographical references and index.
    ISBN 978-0-89281-368-1
    1. Tantrism. 2. Shaktism. 3. Yoga. I. Title.
BL 1238.84.E8613   1992
294.5'514--dc20   92-5008
                                                            CIP

Printed and bound in the United States

20   19   18   17   16   15   14   13

Text design by Charlotte Tyler

CONTENTS

TRANSLATOR'S ACKNOWLEDGMENTS

I would like to thank the following people, who have contributed to this translation with their encouragement and technical assistance:

• My father, who first taught me English as a child, for finding the time and the patience to assist me in the translation of the Conclusion. I love you.

• Susan Pitol, for going over the rough edges of some parts of my translation, though she had a busy schedule. Your help was greatly appreciated.

• David Shocklee, Reference Librarian at St. Louis University, for locating and providing me with much-needed interlibrary loans. Your speed and patience with my constant requests makes you, in my eyes, the greatest in your profession.

• Ehud Sperling, president of Inner Traditions, for his commitment to publish and to popularize the controversial thought of Julius Evola. You are an anticonformist, an open-minded thinker, and a courageous publisher.

• Larry Hamberlin, for providing good insights and doing a great editing job. You know your subject matter inside and out.

*I wish to dedicate this translation
to my two lovely daughters,
Giuliana and Michela.*

TRANSLATOR'S INTRODUCTION

The name of the Italian thinker Julius Evola (1898–1974) is virtually
unknown within the American academic community. To the best of
my knowledge, only two American scholars have so far analyzed
Evola's thought: Thomas Sheehan, who first wrote about him from
a philosophical perspective, and Richard Drake, who wrote from a
political and historical perspective.[1]

Considering both the remarkable consistency and *spissitudo
spiritualis* of Evola's thought, and the revival of interest his work
has enjoyed in Europe during the past decade, much work needs to
be done in North America to bridge this cultural gap. My modest
contribution to the popularization of Julius Evola will be limited
here to the religious and spiritual implications of his worldview,
which so far have been neglected by critics and supporters alike,
eager as they are to focus on the political and ideological ramifica-
tions of his thought.

Giulio Cesare Andrea Evola was born in Rome on May 19,
1898, to a noble Sicilian family. During his adolescence, while pursuing a high school diploma in industrial engineering, he developed a keen interest in contemporary literature and art. As he
recalled in his intellectual autobiography, *Il cammino del cinabro*
[1963, 1972, The cinnabar's journey], his favorite pastimes consisted
of painting, one of his natural talents, and of visiting the library as
often as he could, in order to read works by Oscar Wilde, Friedrich
Nietzsche, and Otto Weininger.

When Italy, following the outbreak of World War I, declared war against its former allies Germany and Austria-Hungary, Evola, who did not appreciate this "betrayal," wrote a bold article in a Roman newspaper suggesting that Italy's participation in the war should not have been dictated by nationalistic, democratic, or irredentist concerns. Its publication marked the beginning of Evola's career as an antidemocratic and nonconformist writer.

At the age of nineteen Evola joined the army and participated in the conflict as a mountain artillery officer. An existing photo shows him in his impeccable uniform, with an aristocratically nonchalant look on his face, while on duty at the front on the Asiago plateau, in northern Italy. Though he admitted that he was never involved in significant military operations, his experiences in that mountainous environment, such as climbing, the inner feelings during the ascent, the silence and solitude of the peaks, and the bird's-eye view of the valleys below, made a deep and long-lasting impression on him. He wrote several essays between 1930 and 1942 on what he called the "mystical dimension" of mountain climbing.[2] He also gave instructions that, after his death, the ashes of his cremated body be dispersed from the top of a mountain. A team of disciples, led by two local guides, buried them instead in a glacier on Monte Rosa, forty-two hundred meters above sea level.

The first few years of Evola's life following the end of the war were characterized by spiritual restlessness and by an intense search for an ideological self-identity. Evola began a personal quest for ultimate transcendence, which he believed could be found beyond the ethical and spiritual limitations of bourgeois prejudices. That quest, characterized by Evola's contempt for what is "all too human" (to use an expression dear to Nietzsche) and for daily routines, led him first to dada, the artistic avant-garde movement founded in Zurich by the Romanian artist Tristan Tzara. Thus Evola became a chief representative of the short-lived, canon-breaking Italian dadaist experience. One of his oil paintings of this period, *Inner Landscape, 10:30 a.m.,* is hanging today on a wall of the National Gallery of Modern Art in Rome.

At this time his quest led him also to experiment with hallucinogenic drugs. His longing for the Absolute, for radically intense feelings, for what the Germans call *mehr als leben,* ("more than living")[3] which was frustrated by the contingency of human experience, almost induced him, at the age of twenty-three, to commit suicide. Evola credited his recovery from this apparent manic-depressive syndrome to an ancient Theravadin text, the *Majjhima-*

Nikaya, which had been translated into Italian from Pali by two scholars between 1915 and 1920. In that text he learned that Buddha taught the importance of detachment from one's sensory perceptions and feelings, and even from one's passionate yearning for extinction.[4] The book became one of Evola's favorites. Twenty years later he employed it as the main primary source when writing *La dottrina del risveglio* (1943; [The doctrine of the awakening, 1951]), a book expounding early Buddhist doctrines. Today a copy of this text is found on the shelves of the Indian Institute in Oxford, England, an implicit acknowledgment of its scholarly merits.[5] This text was also instrumental in Osbert Moore's (1905–1960) conversion to Buddhism. Moore, who took the name Nyanamoli Bhikkhu, became a celebrated Pali scholar and translated several Theravadin texts into English.

Between 1923 and 1927 Evola divided his time between the university and an intense schedule of readings in post-Kantian idealist philosophy. He almost completed his undergraduate studies in engineering, but stopped short of getting a degree because of his dislike of academic titles.[6] He also learned German in order to be able to read Schelling and Hegel in the original texts, while systematizing his own philosophical insights, which were inspired by Nietzsche, Max Stirner, Novalis, Michaelstaedter, and the French personalists. During this period he wrote *Saggi sull'idealismo magico* [1925; Essays on magic idealism], *L'individuo ed il divenire del mondo* [1926; The individual and the becoming of the world], *Teoria dell'individuo assoluto* [1927; Theory of the absolute individual], and *Fenomenologia dell' individuo assoluto* [1930; Phenomenology of the absolute individual].[7] In these works Evola adopted the categories of freedom, action and will as his main hermeneutical tools. He also took issue with both realism, which posits the objective existence of the world, and with metaphysical idealism, especially with its Italian trajectories of Benedetto Croce's absolute historicism and of Giovanni Gentile's absolute subjectivism, which see the ego as passive in relation to the world.

Evola's philosophy is based on Arthur Schopenhauer's statement that "the world is my representation," and on Stirner's rejection of entities such as "God" and "humanity."[8] Evola's vision is one of an unlimited independence from any authority other or higher than the Self. He did not hesitate to espouse an epistemological solipsism (though he rejected the term as "inadequate")[9] whereby the individual stands alone in a world of *maya,* in which nature, things, and people are nothing but an illusion. He also postulated the experience of a pure Self, which an individual may or may not experience. This Self is conceived as a pure, self-centered being, which is known in Hindu metaphysics as *atman* and in Greek philosophy as *nous*. While according to these systems this Self is an ontologically given reality present in all human beings, according to Evola it is present only conditionally, as a project or as a task to be fulfilled. This was his view of the Absolute Individual (from the Latin *ab-solutus*, "freed from").

Following these philosophical works, Evola turned his interest elsewhere. In *La Tradizione ermetica* [1931; The hermetic tradition], which according to some should be regarded as the apex of his writing career, Evola expounded the inner and esoteric core of medieval Hermetic and alchemical doctrines; these form the so-called *ars regia*, which is the end product of pre- and non-Christian spiritual traditions. This work did not go unnoticed by C. G. Jung, who commended it as a "detailed account of Hermetic philosophy." Jung also quoted Evola to support his own contention that "the alchemical *opus* deals in the main not just with chemical experiments as such, but with something resembling psychic processes expressed in pseudo-chemical language."[10]

During the Fascist era Evola was somewhat sympathetic to Mussolini and to Fascist ideology, but his fierce sense of independence and detachment from human affairs and institutions prevented him from becoming a card-carrying member of the Fascist party.[11] Because of his belief in the supremacy of ideas over politics and his advocation of esoteric and traditional views, which at times conflicted with government policy,[12] Evola fell out of favor with powerful government officials, who shut down the biweekly periodical he had founded, *La torre*, which ran only ten issues, from February to June 1930.

Although he criticized the materialistic and crude racism of Nazi Germany and of its Italian epigones, Evola was himself a racist. He published four books outlining his views on the subject, one of which, *Sintesi di dottrina della razza* [1941; Synthesis of a doctrine of race], received Mussolini's enthusiastic endorsement. In these books the author outlined his tripartite anthropology: Each person is composed of body, soul, and spirit. The spirit is the principle that determines one's attitude toward the sacred, destiny, life, and death; it is by far the most important element in humankind. Thus the pursuit of the "spiritual race" should take precedence over the selection of the somatic race, which is determined by the biological laws of genetics, and with which the Nazis were obsessed. Racism was for Evola simply an opportunity to proclaim his antiegalitarian and antirationalistic views; Evola, right or wrong, spurned the idea that all people are created equal and thus enjoy equal dignity and rights.

During World War II Evola often traveled to Germany, where his writings had gained him some popularity, and where he visited with representatives of the Konservativ Revolution, a cultural group, and gave lectures at conferences in various cities. In 1945 he was in Vienna when, as a result of a Soviet air raid on the city, he was wounded in the spinal cord by a shell fragment. He later told a friend that instead of taking to an underground refuge, he had been purposefully walking the deserted streets of the Austrian capital.[13] After spending a year and a half in a local hospital, Evola returned to Italy, destined to spend the rest of his life, a long twenty-nine years, in a wheelchair. Serenely accepting what he called a "minor" handicap, he resumed his contribution to various periodicals and publishing houses.

The last years of his life, which Evola spent in his apartment in Rome, were marked by intense physical pain and discomfort, which he endured with braveness and stoic calm. On June 11, 1974, Evola, feeling his own death approaching, asked to be dressed and to be wheeled to his desk, in front of an open window. He lowered his head, never to lift it up again. He died of a heart attack.

Evola's early contact with the Buddhist philosophy of the Majjhima-Nikaya inspired a deepening interest in Eastern spirituality, an interest he pursued in the 1920s while exploring, and eventually rejecting, European realist and idealist philosophies. His rejection of the passive individual posited in those philosophies, along with his adoption of the categories of will, power, and action as privileged means toward liberation and personal fulfillment, led Evola on a quest for Eastern techniques to strengthen the will, foster the power of concentration, and promote mastery over one's thoughts.

In 1923 Evola wrote the introduction to an Italian translation of the Tao-te Ching, in which he commended the Taoist notions of "immanent transcendence" and "inaction" (*wu wei*). Decio Calvari, president of the Italian Independent Theosophical League, introduced Evola to the study of Tantrism. Soon Evola began a correspondence with the learned British orientalist and divulger of Tantrism Sir John Woodroffe (also known by the pseudonym of Arthur Avalon), whose own works and translations of Tantric texts he amply utilized.

While René Guenon (1886–1951) celebrated Vedanta as the quintessence of Hindu wisdom in his *L'homme et son devenir selon le Vedanta* [1925; Man and his becoming according to Vedanta] and upheld the primacy of contemplation or "knowledge" over action, Evola took a different stance from the one advocated by the French representative of esoteric thought. Taking issue with Guenon's view that spiritual authority ranks higher than royal power, Evola wrote *L'uomo come potenza* [Man as power] in 1925; in the third revised edition (1949), the title was changed to *Lo yoga della potenza* [The yoga of power]. This book represents a link between his speculative works and the rest of his literary production, which focused on traditionalist concerns.

The thesis of the book is that the spiritual and social conditions that characterize the Kali Yuga greatly decrease the effectiveness of purely intellectual, contemplative, and ritual paths. In this age of decadence the only way open to those seeking the great liberation is one of action. Tantrism defined itself as *sadhana-darshana*, namely a system based on practice. Hatha yoga and, more specifically, kunda-lini yoga constitute the psychological and mental training of the Tantrikas seeking liberation. While attacking the stereotype according to which Oriental spiritualities are characterized by an escape from the world (as opposed to those of the West, which allegedly promote vitalism, activism, and the will to power), Evola reaffirmed his belief in the primacy of action by outlining the path followed in Tantrism.

Several decades later, a renowned member of the French Academy, Marguerite Yourcenar, paid homage to *Lo yoga della potenza*. She wrote about "the immense benefit which a receptive reader may gain from an exposition such as Evola's"[14] and concluded that "the study of *The Yoga of Power* is particularly beneficial in a time in which every form of discipline is naively discredited."[15]

Without a doubt, Evola is a controversial figure. During his life he was a nonconformist thinker who never fit any preestablished mold. Posthumously his works have become inspirational to young generations sympathetic to neofascism and in search for an ideological guru.[16] Yet, as I have said, it would hardly do justice to the complexity of his thought to dismiss him as merely a fascist and a racist, without taking a close look at the arguments he employed. Today he remains a significant, though not prominent, figure in the cultural milieu. He is not prominent in the sense that he was never an opinion maker, or somebody whose work greatly influenced either the established academic community or the general public. Neither did Evola seek to communicate or to enter into a dialogue with the mass of his contemporaries. On the contrary, Evola always harbored an aristocratic contempt for the hoi polloi, whether they wore business suits or donned academic garbs. He also refrained from attempts to influence or persuade others.

The unofficial motto of his writing career may well have been taken from one of Buddha's sermons: "One should know approval and disapproval, and having known approval and disapproval, one should neither approve nor disapprove—one should simply teach *dhamma*."[17] The reason for his attitude, that is, for his rejection of discursive thought as a privileged means to arrive at the truth, and therefore of dialogue as a primary form of self-expression, has been clearly recognized by Sheehan:

> What Evola has done is to actualize and exaggerate a tendency that is implicit in all Western philosophies based on the primacy—indeed, the possibility—of an intellectual intuition. He repudiates dialogistic, discursive reasoning *(logos, ratio)*, not because he favors a descent to the irrational, but because he affirms, along with Aristotle, the superiority of the supra-rational.[18]

Evola pointed the way to a steep and solitary path that in my view is still a valid alternative to both the path of *koinonia*—of human fellowship, which contemporary society has been promoting for the past thirty years—and the spiritualized bourgeois individualism promoted by the New Age movement.

It is and will always be difficult to categorize Evola's thought. Was he a representative of European traditionalist thought? a master of esotericism? a *visionnaire foudroyé*? a Gnostic thinker? a neo-pagan? a sage—a "man of knowledge" (to use an expression that Carlos Castaneda employed to characterize Don Juan)? a "perennial philosopher?" All of these labels do partial justice to Evola's multi-faceted and complex thought. For many, myself included, he will remain a "stone guest" in our midst.[19]

Guido Stucco
Department of Theological Studies
St. Louis University
St. Louis, Missouri

THE
MEANING AND ORIGIN
OF THE TANTRAS

In the first few centuries of the Christian era, and in a more marked
way around the fifth century A.D., a peculiar upheaval took place in
the area in which the great Indo-Aryan civilization had grown: the
appearance, development, establishment, and diffusion of a new
spiritual and religious trend, characterized by newer features when
compared with the prevalent motifs of the previous period. This
trend penetrated everywhere and heavily influenced what is generally called Hinduism: it affected yoga schools, post-Upanishadic
speculation, and the cults of Vishnu and Shiva. In Buddhism it gave
rise to a new current, the so-called *Vajrayana* (the "Way of the
Diamond" or "Way of the Thunderbolt"). At last it joined with various forms of popular cults and magic practices on the one hand,
and with strictly esoteric and initiatory teachings on the other.

This new current may be designated as *Tantrism*. In the end it
led to a synthesis of all the main motifs of Hindu spirituality,
finding a particular expression and vindicating its own version of
the metaphysics of history. The terms *Tantra* (a word that often
simply means "treatise," or "exposition," since it is derived from
the root *tan* (which means "to extend" and also "to continue," "to
develop"), and *Agama* (a word designating other texts of the same

1

subject matter) have been understood to mean "what has pro-
ceeded," "that which has come down." The intent was to convey
the idea that Tantrism represents an extension or a further development of those traditional teachings originally found in the Vedas
and later articulated in the Brahmanas, the Upanishads, and the
Puranas. That is why the Tantras have claimed for themselves the
dignity befitting a "fifth Veda," that is, a further revelation beyond
what is found in the traditional four Vedas. To this they added a
reference to the doctrine of the four ages (*yugas*) of the world.[1] It is
claimed that the teachings, rites, and disciplines that would have
been viable in the first age (the Krita or Satya Yuga, the equivalent
of Hesiod's "golden age") are no longer fit for people living in the
following ages, especially in the last age, the "dark age" (Kali Yuga,
the "Iron Age," the "Age of the Wolf" in the Edda). Mankind in
these later ages may find knowledge, a worldview, rituals, and
adequate practices for elevating humans over and beyond their
condition and for overcoming death (*mrityun javate*), not in the
Vedas and in other strictly traditional texts, but rather in the Tantras
and in the Agamas. It is stated therefore that only Tantric practices
based on shakti (*shakti-sadhana*) are suitable and efficacious in our
contemporary age: all the others are considered to be as powerless
as a snake deprived of its poison.[2]

Although Tantrism is far from rejecting ancient wisdom, it is
characterized by a reaction against (1) a hollow and stereotypical
ritualism, (2) mere speculation or contemplation, and (3) any asceticism of a unilateral, mortifying, and penitential nature. It opposes
to contemplation a path of action, of practical realization, and of
direct experience. Its password is practice (*sadhana, abhyasa*).[3] This
runs on the lines of what may be designated the "dry way," resembling the original Buddhist doctrine of the awakening, with its
reaction against a degenerated brahmanism and its dislike of speculations and hollow ritualism.[4] One among the many Tantric texts
remarks rather significantly:

> It is a womanly thing to establish superiority through convinc-
> ing arguments; it is a manly thing to conquer the world through
> one's power. Reasoning, argument, and inference may be the
> work of other schools [shastras]; but the work of the Tantra is
> to accomplish superhuman and divine events through the force
> of their own words of power [mantras].[5]

And also:

> The special virtue of the Tantra lies in its mode of Sadhana. It is
> neither mere worship [upasana] nor prayer. It is not lamenting or
> contrition or repentance before the Deity. It is the Sadhana which
> is the union of Purusha and Prakrti; the Sadhana which joins the
> Male Principle and the Mother Element within the body, and
> strives to make the attributed attributeless. . . . This Sadhana is
> to be performed through the awakening of the forces within the
> body. . . . This is not mere "philosophy," a mere attempt to pon-
> der upon the husks of words, but something which is to be done
> in a thoroughly practical matter. The Tantras say: "Begin prac-
> ticing under the guidance of a good Guru; if you do not obtain
> favorable results immediately, you can freely give it up."[6]

Thus Tantras often employ an analogy taken from medicine:
the efficacy of a doctrine, like a drug, is proved by the results it
produces, and in this particular case, by the siddhis, or powers, that
it grants.[7] Another text says: "Yoga siddhis are not obtained by
wearing yoga garments or by conversation about yoga, but only
through tireless practice. This is the secret of success. There is no
doubt about it."[8]

In the previous quotation referring to the body, another important point was alluded to. The analysis of the last age, the "dark
age" or Kali Yuga, brings to light two essential features. The first is
that mankind living in this age is strictly connected to the body and
cannot prescind from it; therefore, the only way open is not that of
pure detachment (as in early Buddhism and in the many varieties
of yoga) but rather that of knowledge, awakening, and mastery
over secret energies trapped in the body. The second characteristic
is that of the dissolution typical of this age. During the Kali Yuga,
the bull of dharma stands on only one foot (it lost the other three
during the previous three ages). This means that the traditional law
(dharma) is wavering, is reduced to a shadow of its former self, and
seems to be almost succumbing. During Kali Yuga, however, the
goddess Kali, who was asleep in the previous ages, is now fully
awake. I will write at greater length about Kali, a prominent Tantric
goddess, in the following pages; for now, let us say that this symbolism implies that during the last age elementary, infernal, and
even abyssal forces are untrammeled. The immediate task consists

3

in facing and absorbing these forces, in taking the risk of "riding the tiger," to use a Chinese expression that may best describe this situation, or "to transform the poison into medicine," according to a Tantric expression. Hence the rituals and special practices of what has been named Left-Hand Tantrism, or the Path of the Left Hand (Vama-marga), which despite some problematic aspects (orgies, use of sex, etc.) represents one of the most interesting forms within the trend analyzed in this study.

It is therefore stated—and this is significant—that considering the situation of the Kali Yuga, teachings that were previously kept secret may now be revealed in different degrees, though a word of caution is issued concerning the danger they may represent for those who are not initiated.[9] Hence what we have so far mentioned: the emergence, in Tantrism, of esoteric and initiatory teachings.

A third point must be emphasized. In Tantrism the passage from the ideal of "liberation" to that of "freedom" marks an essential change in the ideals and ethics of Hinduism. It is true that even previously the ideal of the *jivanmukta* had been known. The word means "one who is freed," that is, the one who has achieved the unconditioned, the *sahaja*, while alive, in his own body. Tantrism introduces a specification, however: to the existential condition of mankind living in the last age, it relates the overcoming of the antithesis between enjoyment of the world and ascesis, or yoga, which is spiritual discipline aimed at liberation. "In the other schools—thus claim the Tantras—one excludes the other, but in the path we follow these opposites meet."[10] In other words, a discipline is developed that allows one to be free and invulnerable even while enjoying the world, or anything the world may offer. In the meantime, the world ceases to be seen in terms of *maya*—that is, pure appearance, illusion, or mirage—as is the case in Vedantic philosophy. The world is not maya but power. This paradoxical coexistence of freedom, or of the dimension of transcendence in one's self, and enjoyment of the world, of freely experimenting with the world's pleasures, carries the strictest relation with Tantrism's formula and main goal: the union of the impassive Shiva with the ardent Shakti in one's being and at all levels of reality.

This leads us to consider a further fundamental element of Tantrism, namely, Shaktism. In the complex movement called Tantrism, a central role was played by the emergence and predominance of the figure and of the symbol of a goddess or divine woman, Shakti, in its various epiphanies (especially under the forms of Kali and Durga). She may be either portrayed by herself, as the supreme principle of the universe, or reproduced under the species of multiple Shaktis, that is, female divinities who accompany male Hindu gods (who had enjoyed a greater autonomy in the previous era), and even various buddhas and bodhisattvas of late Buddhism. This marks the emergence in a thousand forms of the motif of divine couples, in which the feminine, Shaktic element enjoys a great role, to the point of becoming the predominant element in some of its currents.

Strictly speaking, this current (Shaktism) has archaic exogenous origins, and it traces its roots to an autochthonous spirituality that is visibly analogous to that of the protohistoric, pelasgic, and pre-Hellenic Mediterranean world; in fact, the Hindu "black goddesses" (such as Kali and Durga) and those worshiped in paleo-Mediterranean areas (Demeter Melaina, Cybele, Diana of Ephesus, and Diana of Tauris, including their Christian counterparts such as the "black Madonnas" and Saint Melaina) can be reduced to the same prototype. In this substratum, corresponding to India's Dravidian populations and, in part, to strata and cycles of older civilizations, such as that which was brought to light in various excavation sites at Mohenjo-Daro and Harappa (dating from 3000 B.C.), the cult of a Great Mother or Universal Mother (*magna mater*) was a central motif, and it recovered an importance practically unknown to the Aryan-Vedic tradition and to its essentially virile and patriarchical spirituality. This cult, which during the Aryan (Indo-European) conquest and colonization survived by going underground, reemerged in Tantrism, in the manifold variety of Shaktic Hindu and Tibetan divinities. The result was, on the one hand, the revivifying of what had been latent in popular classes and, on the other hand, the outlining of a Tantric worldview.

Metaphysically speaking, the divine couple corresponds to the two essential aspects of every cosmic principle: the god representing the unchanging dimension, the goddess representing the energy, the acting power of phenomena, and in a sense the dimension of immanence ("life" versus "being"). The appearance of Shaktism in the ancient Indo-Aryan world during the Kali Yuga may be considered a barometric sign of a shifting of perspectives; it speaks of an interest in "immanent" and active principles at work in the world, rather than of anything related to sheer transcendence.

Besides, the name of the goddess, Shakti, comes from the root *shak* ("to be able to," "to have the strength to act"), which means "power." On a speculative note, we may add that the view of the world that identifies in Shakti the supreme principle is also a view

5

of the world as power. More so than others, the Tantrism of the Kashmir school, by associating this view to traditional speculations and by reformulating on this foundation the theory of cosmic principles (*tattva*) typical of Sankhya and the other darshanas, was responsible for developing a metaphysical synthesis of great value, more on which will be found later, and which constitutes the general background for the entire system of Tantric yoga and related disciplines. Here Shakti has almost completely lost her original maternal and gynocratic features and has assumed the metaphysical features of the primordial principle, thus becoming closely related to Upanishadic or Mahayana Buddhist doctrines, which derived from that principle a specifically activistic and energetic emphasis.

It is also understandable how Shaktism and Tantrism contributed, in Hindu and Tibetan areas, to the development of magical practices, often of an inferior kind, which bordered on witchcraft; eventually, what frequently took place was a reviviscence of practices and rituals proper of the previously mentioned pre-Indo-European substratum. As we shall see, however, these very same practices, often of an orgiastic and sexual nature, did not fail, in a Tantric milieu, to rise to a higher plane.

As for the rest, the various goddesses, modifications of the one Shakti, were differentiated in two kinds: the first, luminous and beneficial (e.g., Parvati, Uma, Lakshiami, Gauri); the second, frightful and dark, (Kali, Durga Bhairavi, Camunda). This differentiation is not precise, since the same goddess could assume either of the two aspects when reflecting the attitude of the devotee approaching her. In any event, the goddesses of the bright and prevalently maternal kind, who preserved their pre-Aryan nature, have become pivotal in those popular and devotional religious movements paralleling Tantrism, which shared with Tantrism an intolerance for a stereotypical ritualism and for mere speculation. People turned to devotion and to cult (*bhakti* and *puja*), in order to achieve emotional experiences (*rasa*) with mystical overtones. The natural consequence of this was that the Goddess in her bright aspect became the favorite reference point of the masses, coming to hold almost the same status that the "Mother of God" enjoys in Christian devotion. It must be noticed that this orientation was not a new phenomenon, since one of its roots was Vaishnavism (the cult of Vishnu). What was new, however, almost having the value of a barometric index, was its development and diffusion outside the lower classes of Indian society, to which it had so far been confined, and its blossoming into the so-called Way of Devotion, Bhaktimarga, which had in Ramanuja its chief representative. I have commented elsewhere on the analogies with Christian theism.[11]

The properly Tantric goddesses, however, are the Shaktis of the Path of the Left Hand, mainly Kali and Durga. Under their aegis Tantrism becomes integrated with Shaivism, the cult of Shiva, while through the bright goddesses it encounters Vaishnavism and the Way of the Right Hand. It is claimed that even Shiva has no Vedic origins: in the Vedas one finds Rudra, who may be considered his equivalent, and who propitiated Shiva's reception in the Hindu pantheon. Rudra, the "Lord of Thunder," is a personification of the divinity in its destructive aspect, that of a "destructive transcendence"; therefore, in more practical terms he is the "god of death," the "slayer." Shaivism exalts Shiva, the embodiment of all the attributes of the supreme deity, as well as the creator portrayed in an awesome and highly symbolical icon, Nataraja, which is his dance representing the rhythm of both the creation and destruction of the worlds. In a Tantric context, Shiva, while preserving the features typical of pure transcendence, is usually associated with a terrifying Shakti, such as Kali and Durga, who personify his own unrestrained and untamable manifestation. When Hinduism canonized the doctrine of *trimurti* (i.e., the three aspects of the one supreme principle, personified in three divinities, Brahma, Vishnu, and Shiva), the meaning of the two ways, the Right Hand and Left Hand, became clear. The first element in the trimurti is Brahma, the creator god; the second is Vishnu, the god preserving creation and the cosmic order; and the third is Shiva, the destroyer (as a result of his transcendence acting on what is finite and conditioned). The Way of the Right Hand is under the aegis of the first two gods, or aspects of the divine, while the Path of the Left Hand is under the sign of the third God, Shiva. This is the way that essentially emerged from the encounter between Shaivism and Tantrism.

Summing up, we may consider typical of Tantric speculation a metaphysics and a theology of *shakti*, namely, of the Principle as power, or of the "active brahman." What comes next is the use of sadhana, the practice leading to self-realization. Together with the metaphysics of shakti, we find an emphasis on the magical and empowering dimensions within a vast traditional and ritualistic heritage, which often led to the formulation of esoteric and initiatory teachings. In particular, the doctrine of the mantras, which evolved from a metaphysics of the word, was assimilated to Tantrism. The mantra came to be seen no longer primarily as a liturgical formula, prayer, or mystical sound, but rather as "word of power," gaining such an importance that Tantrism was sometimes referred to (especially in some questionable Tibetan Buddhist versions) as Mantrayana, the Way of Mantras. Practical concerns led to a strict connection between Tantrism and yoga. A specifically Tantric character is found particularly in hatha yoga (the "violent" yoga, for such is the literal meaning of the word, and not "physical" yoga or, even worse, the "yoga of health"), understood as "yoga of the serpent's power," kundalini yoga, which is based on the awakening and employment, in view of one's liberation, of the primordial shakti immanent in the human organism. In this kind of yoga we find a science of the "occult corporeity," that is, the hyperphysical anatomy and physiology of the human organism, in the context of correlations between man and world, microcosm and macrocosm. Breathing and sex are considered to be the only two disciplines still available to mankind living in the Kali-Yuga. Sadhana is based on them. In yoga, strictly speaking, which carried on the vast majority of Patañjali's classical yoga, the emphasis is mainly on breathing, *pranayama*. Women, sex, and sexual magic play a major role in another sector of Tantrism in which, as it was already mentioned, even ancient practices of the dark pre-Aryan substratum were borrowed, transformed, integrated, and elevated to an initiatory plane. Especially in Siddhantachara and in Kulachara, considered by authoritative texts such as the Kularnava-Tantra (11, 7, 8) and the Mahanirvana-Tantra (4:43–45, 15:179–80) to be the two highest and most esoteric schools of the Path of the Left Hand, the emphasis shifted from liberation to the freedom of the man-god, that is, one who has overcome the human condition and is beyond any law. The highest concern in this current is how to achieve the supreme state that is seen as the union of Shiva and Shakti, whose mating symbolizes the impulse of reuniting being (Shiva) with power (Shakti). Tantric Buddhism saw in the achievement of this unity the so-called *mahasukhakaya*, a "body" or a condition even higher than the *dharmakaya* itself, which is the cosmic root from which every awakened one, or buddha, derives.[12]

Recently Tantrism has become well known in the West, and its importance within Hinduism acknowledged. Besides some scholarly monographs, the merit of acquainting the Western world with a vast material of texts and translations concerning Hindu Tantrism belongs to Sir John Woodroffe (Arthur Avalon is a pseudonym that he used when writing books together with Hindu scholars).[13] W. Y.

Evans-Wentz and the Lama Kazi Dawa-Samdup are responsible for the translation of various texts of Tantric and Tibetan Buddhism, the so-called Vajrayana, that previously existed only in the form of codices and manuscripts.[14] One should also mention the pioneering works of De la Vallee Poussin, of Von Glasenapp, G. Tucci, and H. Hoffmann, and especially the precious material concerning Tantrism in Mircea Eliade's superb work *Yoga: Immortalité et liberté* (Paris, 1954). Previously, outside the specialized circles of learned orientalists, Tantrism was relatively unknown and even portrayed under a sinister light (someone even referred to it as "the worst kind of black magic"). This happened because what had been known was considered excesses or deviations from this current, instead of authentic elements that clashed with the puritanical and "spiritualist" mentality of the time, thus causing scandals and outrage.

This presentation, in which I have tried to quote the original texts as often as possible (especially those published by Woodroffe), deals essentially with doctrinal and practical aspects of Tantrism. I have noticed that Tantrism appears to be a synthesis, or better, a supplement of previous teachings. I will therefore expound many of those teachings that were incorporated in Tantrism, so that this book may also provide the reader with an overview of Hindu tradition, although mainly from a Tantric perspective.

I have resolved not to add anything personal or arbitrary; however, since my task is not merely to expound but also to interpret esoteric knowledge, which in Tantrism plays a major role, I have been able to substantiate some elements, owing to my ability to read between the lines of the texts, my personal experiences, and the comparisons I have established with parallel teachings found in other esoteric traditions. As for the methodological principle adopted in this book, I have adopted the guiding principle employed in my previous books: to maintain the same distance both from the two-dimensional, specialized findings typical of university-level and academic orientalism and from the digressions of our contemporary "spiritualists" and "occultists."

KNOWLEDGE AND POWER

Tantrism, in its emphasis on self-empowerment, recaptures and stresses what may be called "traditional knowledge" of a metaphysical rather than profane nature. This knowledge is witnessed from the very beginning not only in Hindu areas but also in other traditional civilizations of a higher kind, such as those that flourished before the advent of modern civilization. It will be useful to point out briefly the implications of this kind of knowledge.

India possessed a metaphysics based on "revelation" (*akachani,* *shruti*), a term that should be understood differently than in the context of monotheistic religions, in which it is assumed that the deity has bestowed special knowledge on humanity, who is thus a passive recipient, and that a given organization (e.g., the Christian church) is in charge of safeguarding divine revelation in the form of dogmas.

Shruti, however, corresponds to the exposition of what has been "seen" and revealed (made known) by certain individuals, the so-called *rishi,* whose high "stature" is at the basis of tradition. *Rishi,* from *dric,* "to see," means precisely "one who has seen." The Vedas, which are considered to be the foundation of the entire orthodox Hindu tradition, take their name from the word *vid,* meaning both "to see" and "to know," which is an eminent and direct kind of knowledge assimilated by analogy to the act of seeing. The ancient Western counterpart to this term is found in Hellas, where the notion of "idea," because of its root *id*, identical to the Sanskrit *vid* (hence *Veda*), suggests a knowledge based on seeing. Tradition in the form of shruti records and proposes what the rishi have "seen" directly, on a superindividual and superhuman plane. In its inner and essential aspect, the foundation of the entire Hindu metaphysics may be said to rest on this.

Regarding a knowledge that presents itself under these terms, the attitude to be taken is not different from that taken toward one who claims that in an unknown continent there are certain things, or toward a physicist expounding the results of his experiments. One may simply believe, relying on the authority and truthfulness of the interlocutor; or one may attempt to verify personally whether what has been said is true or not, in the first instance, by undertaking a trip, and in the second, by gathering all the elements necessary for reproducing the experiment oneself. These are the only two sensible attitudes to be taken regarding a rishi's claims, unless one intends to ignore anything related to metaphysics. This is not a matter of abstract concepts, of "philosophy" in the modern sense of the term, or of dogmas, but rather of material from which experiences can be derived, since tradition offers the means and singles out the disciplines with which it is possible to "verify," through personal and direct evidence, the reality of what has been communicated. It seems that in the Christian West the adoption of a similar experimental approach has been granted only to mysticism, since theology defined it as a *cognitio experimentalis dei* and described it as something that is beyond both mere faith and agnosticism. (Christian mysticism, however, should not be equated with the kind of knowledge I have been talking about, because its background is emotional rather than noetic, and religious rather than metaphysical).

The prevailing orientation of the Tantras runs on the same lines. They repeatedly affirm that a mere theoretical exposition of doctrine has no value whatsoever. What especially matters, according to them, is the practical method of self-fulfillment, the body of means and rituals through which certain hidden truths may be recognized. This is why Tantras wish to be referred to as *sadhana-shastra*—sadhana being derived from the root *sadh*, which means exerting will power, effort, training, or activity in the hope of achieving a given result. A Tantric author remarked: "At the present time the general public are ignorant of the principles of the Tantra

Sastra. The cause of this ignorance is the fact that the Tantra Sastra is a Sadhana Sastra, the greater part of which becomes intelligible only through Sadhana."[1]

It is therefore not enough to abide by the theory of the identity between the deeper self (*atman*) and the principle of the universe (*brahman*) and "to remain idle, vaguely thinking of the conscious ether." The Tantras deny the value of knowledge to this. In order to obtain true knowledge, one must be transformed by action; hence *kriya*, action, became the password.[2] To this idea, Tantric Buddhism, or Vajrayana, gave a supple expression by employing the symbol of sexual union between the "effective way" (*upaya*) and knowing, in which the former plays the male role.

It should be noted that in the higher forms of Tantrism this point of view is even applied to cult and eventually not only to metaphysics, to the sacred and transforming knowledge, but also to knowledge of nature.

As far as cult (puja) is concerned, I shall discuss later the special role that it plays in Tantrism, together with the various evocations and ritual and magical identifications. Moreover, it is a Tantric notion that one cannot adore a god without "becoming" that god,[3] which brings us back to experimentalism rather than to any religious dualism.

As far as the sciences of nature are concerned, we would have to go to great lengths to explain the opposition between "traditional" knowledge and knowledge of the so-called scientific, modern type. This is not just the view of Tantrism, since on this matter it followed previous traditions and in the process of developing its own cosmology and its doctrine of manifestation it borrowed, adapted, and developed their teachings and fundamental principles.

Briefly stated, here is the situation: According to the modern point of view (which in a Hindu perspective would be considered to be typical of the most advanced phase of the "dark age"), we can directly apprehend reality only through those aspects revealed to us by physical senses and by their extension, namely scientific instruments, or, according to the terminology proper to some philosophies, through its "phenomenic aspects." Positive sciences gather and organize data provided by sensory experiences, and only after having made a certain choice between them (excluding those with a qualitative character and essentially relying on those that are susceptible to measurement and "computation") does it inductively arrive at some knowledge and laws of an abstract and conceptual nature. To them, however, there no longer corresponds an intuition, an unmediated perception, or an intrinsic evidence. Their truth is indirect and conditioned, and it depends on experimental examination, which may eventually lead to a reshaping of the previous system.

In the modern world, in addition to science one encounters "philosophy," but only to find in it abstractions and a mere conceptual speculation, which is broken down into a discordant multiplicity of systems espoused by individual thinkers. This world of philosophy may be said to be eminently "unrealistic." The choice seems to be between these two alternatives: either a direct and concrete knowledge depending on the senses, or a knowledge that is presumed to be able to go beyond this "phenomenic" world of appearances, but that is still abstract, cerebral, merely conceptual, or hypothetical (scientific philosophies and theories).

This means that the ideal of "seeing," namely, of a direct form of knowledge verging on the heart of reality, despite having a noetic, objective character (an ideal that was still preserved in the medieval notion of *intuitio intellectualis*), has been set aside. It is interesting to notice that in the so-called European critical philosophy of Kant, intellectual intuition is still thought of as a faculty capable of apprehending not just the phenomena but the essences as well (the "thing in itself," the noumenon), and yet this capability is assumed to be precluded to man (just as scholastic philosophy had taught). That assumption was made in order to clarify, through antithesis, what according to Kant was the only knowledge available to man: mere sensory knowledge, scientific knowledge, whose abstract, nonintuitive character we have so far discussed, and which may show with a high degree of precision how forces of nature act, but not what they are.

In esoteric teachings, including the Hindu ones, such a limitation is considered to be surmountable. As we shall see, classical yoga in its various articulations (*yoganga*) may be said to offer the methods of a systematic overcoming of such a limitation. The bottom line is this: there is no such thing as a world of "phenomena," of perceptible forms, and behind it, an impenetrable, true reality: the essence. There is only one given reality, which is multidimensional; there is also a hierarchy of possible forms of human and superhuman experiences, in relation to which these various dimensions are progressively disclosed, until one is able to perceive directly the essential reality. The type or ideal of knowing, which is that of a direct knowledge (*sakshastra, aparokshajnana*) of a real experience and of an immediate evidence (*anubhava*), is always preserved in all these levels. As we previously stated, the common person, especially the one living in the end times, in the Kali Yuga, can enjoy such a knowledge only when it comes to physical and sensory reality. The rishi, the yogi, or the Tantric siddha can go beyond that reality, in the context of what may be called an integral and transcendental experimentalism. According to this point of view there is no such thing as a relative reality and, beyond it, an absolute, impervious reality, but rather a relative, conditioned method of perceiving the only reality, and an absolute method.

The immediate connection between this traditional epistemology and the main concerns of Tantrism is rather obvious. In fact, in this order of ideas, the way to any superior knowledge seems to be contingent upon one's self-transformation, an existential and ontological change of level, and therefore, upon action, sadhana. This conception contrasts with the general view offered by the modern world. Modern scientific knowledge, in its technical applications, confers to modern man multiple possibilities with impressive consequences on the practical and material plane, while leaving him, on a concrete plane, at the same level. For instance, if through modern science we happen to learn the approximate processes and constant laws of physical phenomena, our existential situation has still not changed a bit. In the first place, the fundamental elements of physics are nothing but differential functions and integrals, namely, abstract algebraic entities, of which, in a strict sense, we cannot claim to have either an intuitive image or a concept, since they are mere instruments of calculation ("energy," "mass," "cosmic constant," "curved space," are nothing but verbal symbols). Second, after we have "known" all this, our real relationship with phenomena still has not changed. The same applies to the scientist who elaborates knowledge of such a kind and even to one who develops innovative technology: fire will still burn him, organic modifications and passions will still trouble his soul, time will still dominate him with its laws, the sight of nature will still not speak to him, but it will mean to him less than it did to primitive man. This is because the scientific formation of modern civilized man entirely desacralizes the world and petrifies it in the ghost of sheer, mute appearances. These appearances, along with knowledge of the kind discussed so far, make room only for the aesthetic and lyrical emotions of poets and artists, which obviously have no scientific or metaphysical value, being merely subjective experiences.

The prevalent alibi of modern science is the claim to power; and that argument, in this context, deserves to be considered, since shakti as power, as well as *siddhis* (namely, powers), plays an important role in Tantrism and related currents. Modern science offers the proof of its validity through the positive results achieved, particularly by putting at man's disposal such a power that has, so it is claimed, no precedents in previous civilizations.

We are dealing here with a misconception of the term *power*, since no distinction is made between a relative, external, inorganic, conditioned power and true power. Obviously, all the opportunities offered by science and technology to people of the Kali Yuga are exclusively of the first type. Action produces results only because it conforms itself to given laws, which scientific research has pointed out, laws that action presupposes and obeys to the letter. The effect, therefore, is not directly connected to man, to the Self, or to his free will, as to its cause; between action and result there is a series of intermediaries that do not depend on the Self, and that are necessary in order to achieve what one wants. It is not just a matter of devices and machines, but of laws, of natural determinism that could go this way or that way, unintelligible in its essence; such mechanical power, is, after all, precarious.

In no way does it represent a possession of the Self, nor is it one of the Self's powers. What has been said about scientific knowledge applies as well: it does not change the human condition, the existential situation of an individual, nor does it presuppose or require any transformation of that kind. It is rather something added on, superimposed, which does not imply any self-transformation. No one claims that we show any real superiority when we are capable of doing this or that by availing ourselves of any technical means: we do not cease to be mere humans, not even as lords of atomic weapons who can disintegrate a planet by pushing a button. And worse yet, if as a consequence of any given cataclysm people living in the Kali Yuga were deprived of all their machines, in the greatest majority of cases they would probably find themselves in a worse predicament than uncivilized primitives do when facing the forces of nature and the elements. That is because machines and technology have atrophied their true strength. We may well say that modern man, by virtue of a diabolical mirage, has been seduced by the "power" he has at his disposal, and of which he is so very proud.

That which does not depend on the laws of nature, but which rather bends, changes, and suspends them, is a different kind of power. It is a direct acquisition of a few superior beings. The condition for such power and for the real knowledge I previously mentioned lies in the removal of the human condition, that is, of the limit represented by what the Hindus call "physical Self" (*bhutatman*, the elemental Self). The axiom of all yoga, of Tantric sadhana and analogous disciplines, corresponds to Nietzsche's saying "man is something that must be overcome," only taken more seriously. As is the case with initiation in a general sense, the human condition is not accepted as one's final destiny; it is intolerable to be merely mortal. Overcoming the human condition, in the framework of such disciplines, is in various degrees the condition for authentic power, for the acquisition of siddhis. To be precise, these siddhis do not represent the goal (to consider them as such is often reputed to be a deflection), but rather they are the natural consequence of an achieved superior existential and ontological status. Far from being something added on or extrinsic, they are a characteristic of a spiritual superiority (it is interesting to notice that the term *siddhis*, besides "extraordinary powers," means "perfections"). Therefore, they are always a personal achievement, and as such they cannot be transferred, nor are they "democratizable."

There is a deep hiatus separating the traditional and the modern world. The knowledge and powers pursued by the modern world are democratic, that is, available to anyone endowed with enough intelligence to achieve, through educational institutions, a knowledge of modern natural sciences. It is enough to gain through training a certain level of knowledge that does not involve the deepest nucleus of one's being in order to be able to correctly deploy technological means. A handgun will produce the same results in the hands of a lunatic, a soldier, or a great statesman; in the same sense, anyone can be transported in a few hours from one continent to another. We may well say that this "democracy" has been the leading principle in the systematic organization of modern science and technology. As we have seen, the real differentiation of beings is the condition for an inalienable knowledge and power, which cannot be transferred to others; they are exclusive and "esoteric," not artificially, but by virtue of their very nature. They represent exceptional peaks of achievement of which the whole of society cannot partake. What is open to society are only opportunities of an inferior kind, precisely those that have been developed in the late Kali Yuga, in a civilization that has no correspondence with previous ones. In the context of traditional civilizations, besides these material opportunities (the paucity of which was due to the lack of interest people had in them),[4] artistic activities could be pursued by anyone who had any interest in them. Generally speaking, they were characterized by various ways of life essentially oriented toward higher planes of being. This spiritual climate has been maintained in more than one area until relatively recent times.

I thought it necessary, as a way of introduction, to expose these critical and theoretical principles in order to give the reader a sense of direction into the spiritual world we are about to enter. As we approach our subject matter, I will add two more considerations, the first, again, concerning the science of nature. As I have said, in the data furnished by common experience, modern science has found only the so-called first qualities, namely, extension and movement, to be useful for its own purposes. The so-called secondary qualities, such as the quality of things and phenomena, have been excluded as such and treated only from a psychological and subjective point of view. In reality, however, no object or phenomenon is directly experienced through extension and movement only, but is rather perceived together with other qualities. In India, a qualitative-psychological physics has been developed, with "atoms" and "elements" that consider reality not merely under the species of extension and movement but rather according to various qualities corresponding to different senses; such are the *mahabhuta*, the *paramanu*, and the *tanmantra*. These principles of the natural order are not abstract speculations but rather potential objects of a direct experience, while at the same time they retain the value of explanatory principles of the system on which the world is built. They can be perceived by the special faculties developed by yoga and by sadhana. Then we can see how there corresponds to them a meaning, a form of evidence or special enlightenment.

The perfect, liminal degree, in higher knowledge, is that in which being is identified with knowing, in which the contraposition between subject and object, between I and not-I (which is found in every form of modern scientific knowledge, constituting its methodological premise) is finally removed. Jnana yoga, in its last stage, aims at achieving this state, called *samadhi*. But if instead of turning to Patañjali's Yoga-Sutras we turn to Tantric metaphysics, the essence or bottom line of everything is shakti, or power; hence the connection with the doctrine of siddhis, of superhuman powers. We can also read in it about an alleged process in the world in which Shakti, after becoming explicit in the realm of the not-I and consequently becoming obfuscated and unconscious, gradually awakens, acquires a conscious form (*chidrupini-shakti*), unites with her principle or "male partner" (Shiva), and finally becomes one with him. As we shall see, according to Tantric hatha yoga, this process is repeated inside the practitioner. It forms the basis of a doctrine of certainty.

A Tantric commentator remarks that things are power and the "power of a thing does not wait for intellectual recognition." One may amuse oneself by calling the world an illusion, or think of it as unreal, but "karma, the force of action, will force him to believe in it." We can always ask of something, Why is it like this and not like something else? "In reality the Lord himself [Ishvara], would not elude these questions, which are the natural mark of ignorance."[5] These problems come up as long as one remains in an extraneous or passive relationship with Shakti's manifestations in the world. These problems end, the Tantric author claims, only when the individual, because of sadhana, activates in himself the Shiva principle, that is, the radiant and dominating counterpart of the primeval power. In him, there will then emerge a particular and suprarational kind of evidence and certainty, bound to a power. It is claimed concerning the fundamental requirement of practice: "Every Scripture is but a means. It is not useful to one who has not yet known the Devi [goddess = Shakti] and is not useful to one who has already known her."[6] After all, it is an Upanishadic theme that "into blind darkness enter they that worship ignorance; into darkness greater than that, as it were, they that delight in knowledge," and that those who have studied, upon attaining true knowledge, "throw away books as if they were on fire."[7]

The abovementioned polemical remark against those who think of the world as illusion was obviously aimed at that current of thought whose most extreme expression was represented by the Vedantic doctrine of Shankara. It is not meaningless, at this point, to see how that polemic was conducted. Vedanta claims that the only reality is that of the plain Absolute, in its formless and undetermined aspect, the so-called *nirguna-brahman*. Everything else, the world and all its manifestations, is "false," a mere product of the imagination (*kalpana*), a mere appearance (*avastu*): here is the well-known and much-abused concept of maya, of the world as maya. A hiatus is thus established: nothing unites the real, *brahman*, with the manifestation, the world. Between them there is not even an antithesis, since one is and the other is not.

In the polemics carried on by the Tantras, their orientation toward concreteness is confirmed. It is true that from the point of view of the Absolute, the manifestation cannot exist in and by itself, since there cannot be a being outside of Being.[8] A question may be asked, however, as to what exactly is one who professes the doctrine of maya: if he is *Brahman* itself or one of the beings that exist in the realm of maya. As long as one remains a human, namely a finite and conditioned being, one certainly cannot be called *nirguna-brahman*, which is the unchanging pure Absolute without determinations and forms. Therefore, such a person cannot be but maya, since outside of *nirguna-brahman* one finds only maya. But if that person—the extremist Vedantist—in his existential reality, as a human, a *jiva*, a living being, is maya, then everything that he claims will be but maya (appearance and falsehood), including his theory according to which only *nirguna-brahman* is real while everything else is illusion and falsehood.[9]

This argument, which employs a subtle dialectic, is unexceptionable. Tantras say that the world as we know it may be maya from the point of view of *brahman* and of the siddha, one who has completely overcome the human condition. But such is not the case from the point of view of every finite consciousness, in the experience of common people, to whom it is instead an indisputable reality that cannot be prescinded from. Until one perseveres in his condition, one is not authorized to call the world maya in the Vedantic sense of the word. In a commentary to the Isha-Upanishad, it is emphasized that by insisting on the doctrine of maya and on the absolute contradiction between the supreme principle and everything that is determined and endowed with form, the very possibility of yoga and of sadhana would be compromised, since "it is impossible that something would be transformed into its own very contradiction."[10]

"We are mind and body: if mind and body (inasmuch as they belong to the world of maya) are false, how can one hope to achieve through them that which is true?"[11] Strictly speaking, the extremist Vedantic doctrine of maya would therefore deny to the individual the very possibility of elevating oneself toward the principle, since such a possibility presupposes that between these two no hiatus exists (a relationship between not-being and being), but rather a certain continuity. That is why, because of its concern to establish the necessary premises of yoga and, generally speaking, of sadhana, the practice leading to realization, and in order to prevent any contemplative escapism, Tantrism formulated a doctrine of the "active *brahman*" that is no less metaphysical than Vedanta's. Tantrism accomplished this by introducing the notion of shakti and by reshaping the maya theory. In the following pages we will mainly deal with that doctrine.

· III ·

SHAKTI:
THE WORLD AS POWER

First of all, let us assess the new form that Tantric metaphysics assumed following the assimilation and transformation into a main hermeneutical principle of the ancient idea of the Devi, or Great Mother, who is conceived as the supreme deity.

The starting point is represented by the acknowledgement that the principle and measure of every real being and form is a multiform energy, an acting power that expresses itself in various ways. It is not a coincidence, as someone remarked, that the German word for reality, *Wirklichkeit*, comes from the verb *wirken*, "to act." This is also the case in Tantric metaphysics. With regard to power (shakti), even what we call "person" occupies an ontologically subordinated rank, including Ishvara, who is the God of theism. This radical version of Shaktism denies the existence of a principle "endowed" with power, yet distinct from it. The argument runs on these lines: "If everything exists in virtue of shakti, why look for its source? You feel the need to identify the principle or support on which shakti is based. Are you not then compelled to explain on what principle shakti foundation is based?"[1]

The similarities between Tantrism and older Hindu metaphysical systems may easily be established as follows: These systems did not stop at the concepts of "being" and "person." The counterpart of being (*sat*) is nonbeing (*asat*). Beyond both of them we find the Absolute (*brahman*, which is neuter, should not be confused with the name Brahma, which is masculine). Hindu metaphysics did not employ a theistic notion of "God," conceived as a person (Ishvara, Brahma, and analogous hypostases), as the ultimate reference point. Rather, *brahman* is something that transcends the personal deity and is thought of in terms of primordial and abyssal energy. The Tantric Shakti eventually came to be identified with it, but in the course of this process she lost all of her specifically feminine traits,[2] since *brahman* is beyond the masculine/feminine differentiation. Shakti also lost the primacy she enjoyed as the feminine element, which is typical of ancient civilizations. That primacy derives from the capability of giving birth and from being thought of, in a cosmic context, as an incubating womb. Generating as well as creating are, however, still considered to be subordinated and partial functions, and Brahma's rather than *brahman's* prerogatives.

Shakti is therefore characterized by the same attributes usually associated with *brahman*; nothing exists outside of her, since she is "one without a second" (*advaya*). All living beings find their origin, life, and purpose in her: "Thou art all power. It is by thy power that we are powerful."[3]

It is also said:

> Shakti is the root of every finite existence. The worlds are her manifestation; she supports them and one day they will be reabsorbed into her. . . . She is the supreme *brahman* (Parabrahman). . . . She is the mother of all the gods; without Shakti they would cease to exist.[4]

She is called Paratpara, "supreme of the supreme,"[5] that is, the *brahman* invoked in Hindu Brahman metaphysical tradition. She is the "eternal energy of him who sustains the universe" (*vaishnavishakti*), and in relation to the *trimurti*, the divine triad of Hinduism, it is said:

> It is by Thy [Shakti's] power only that Brahma creates, Vishnu maintains, and, at the end of things, Shiva destroys the universe. Powerless are they for this but by Thy help. Therefore it is that Thou alone are the Creator, Maintainer, and Destroyer of the world.[6]

And also: "Thou supportest everything, without being supported yourself."[7] Only Shakti is "pure," "naked": "Though having a form, yet thou art always formless."[8]

In this context Shakti is given the name Parashakti, to emphasize that no other being or principle ranks higher than her. The ancient pre-Aryan understanding of Shakti as the *magna mater*, or mother of the gods—a sovereign divinity from whom every life and existence derives—undergoes a radical transformation as a consequence of the encounter with Aryan Upanishadic metaphysics. Shakti there becomes "she who dwells in everything in the form of power" (Shaktirupa).

From the texts we gather a further, particularly relevant element. If we consider the principle of the universe merely in terms of primordial energy, we may be induced to think that its manifestation in the world is nothing but a random, centrifugal movement. That being the case, we would then be reminded of the notion of "life" as it is found in some Western irrationalist philosophies and even in Spinoza's pantheist system. According to Spinoza, the world proceeds eternally and almost necessarily from the substance of the godhead, in the same way that the properties of a triangle derive from its definition. In Tantrism, on the contrary, Shakti's manifestation is considered to be free. Since she is not bound by any external or internal laws, nothing forces her to become apparent: "Thou art power. Who could tell you what to do or not to do?"[9] Since in human experience the ideal prototype of unrestrained action is play (*lila*), the Tantras do not hesitate to call Shakti's manifestation "play" and to say that (1) her essence is play (*lilamayishakti*); (2) her name is "playful," *lalita*;[10] and (3) the supreme Shakti's (Parashakti) solitary game finds expression in every form of manifested and conditioned existence, whether human, subhuman, or divine. Tantric symbolism merged with Shaivist symbols and even appropriated the theme of the dancing god, Nataraja. Dance is something free and uninhibited, representing the unfolding of the manifestation. It is no longer Shiva who engages in the dance, but the goddess Shakti, portrayed with a flaming halo to symbolize her properly productive aspect.

As a natural consequence of this development, the theses of radical Shaktism, which reflected the goddess's ancient sovereignty and ontological priority, were subsequently articulated. This led to the assimilation of Sankhya's metaphysics and to the reappraisal of the maya doctrine during the same period in which Shankara had formulated it.

Sankhya is a darshana[11] based on dualism. As its hermeneutic principle it adopts an original duality, that of *purusha* and *prakriti*, corresponding to the masculine and feminine elements; spirit and nature, and consciousness and unconsciousness. The former is unchangeable, the latter is the principle of movement and of becoming. Sankhya meticulously excluded from the first element, purusha, anything that is not pure, impassive, or action-oriented. Creation derives from a peculiar connection of these two principles and from an action originated by purusha (called "catalysis" in chemistry) and determined just by its presence. The closest analogy I can think of comes from that Aristotelian doctrine which explains the world and its becoming in terms of motion and of the desire awakened in matter (*ule* = prakriti) by the *nous*, or "unmoved mover." Prakriti, as such, is thought of as an equilibrium of three powers (the so-called *gunas*, which I will discuss later). Purusha's reflection on prakriti breaks this equilibrium, and by virtue of an impregnating action it causes motion and thus prakriti's unfolding into the world of forms and phenomena, which is called *samsara*. Sankhya also contemplates a "fallen condition," corresponding to a fundamental notion found in both Hindu and Buddhist metaphysics, namely avidya, or ignorance. Purusha identifies with its own reflection in prakriti, the so-called elemental Self (*bhutatman*), thus forgetting it is "other," that is, the impassive being whose substance is pure light, or the "spectator":

> The immortal soul [*atman*] is like the "drop of water on the lotus leaf." This elemental soul verily is overcome by nature's [prakriti] qualities [gunas]. Now, because of being overcome, he goes on to confusedness; because of confusedness he sees not the blessed Lord [Parabrahman], the causer of action who stands within oneself [*atma-stha*]. Borne along and defiled by the stream of qualities, unsteady, wavering, bewildered, full of desire, distracted, this one goes on to the state of self-conceit (*abhimanatva*). In thinking "This is I" and "That is mine" he binds himself with his self as does a bird with a snare. . . . The person is not overcome. This elemental soul (*bhutatman*) is overcome (*abhibhuta*) because of its attachment to qualities.[12]

Sankhya lent its tenets to classical yoga, which indicated the way leading from prakriti to reintegration with a purely purushic state, which we may call "Olympian," or mukti (release). Yoga pointed the way by promoting detachment from consciousness and from the I (atman = purusha), and by neutralizing those modifica-

23

tions (*vritti*) that are consciously believed to be one's own rather than proper to the other principle (prakriti).

At this point we are not yet dealing with practical applications, but still with cosmological views. Let us proceed. Sankhya offers an explanation of the world, not in terms of pure spirit, or of pure nature, or as being immutable or in a process of becoming, but rather by introducing the purusha-prakriti dyad. These two principles become connected in various ways: following the loss of equilibrium of the gunas, prakriti, after being fertilized by purusha's reflection, "becomes" and grows in the manifested world of "names" and "forms" (*namarupa* is the classical Hindu designation for the differentiated universe).

The Tantric synthesis takes up this paradigm again and reappraises it. Unlike the Sankhya system, purusha and prakriti are no longer conceived as an eternal, primordial duality, but rather as two differentiations or forms of Shakti. Shiva, the personal god now transformed into an impersonal metaphysical principle, corresponds to the former. Shakti corresponds to the latter, though in a limited sense, since she assumes the role of Shiva's counterpart, namely, that of the god's companion and bride; she is also believed to be his power (traditionally the term *shakti* had the meanings of both "power" and "bride"). As it was the case in Sankhya, Shiva retains the attributes of "being," immutability, and the nature of atman, or conscious principle. On her part, Shakti retains the characteristics of movement and mutability. She is the source of productive activities, generation, and vivification. While Sankhya spoke of "reflection" and "action" in terms of pure presence, in the Tantric synthesis the idea of "fertilization" was widely accepted: the union of Shiva and Shakti is believed to generate the universe, with both its static and dynamic components, and with both its immaterial/conscious and material/unconscious forms. The introduction of the purushic, or Shaivist element, discredits the idea that a radical version of Shaktism had upheld instead, namely, that the manifested world is the result of a wild outburst of an undifferentiated, elementary energy.

Hindu Tantric iconography enhanced in various ways the authentic characteristics of the two principles. First, we may recall the icon of Shakti's dance over Shiva's outstretched and still body. In this instance, immobility represents the immutability of the male principle. According to the canons of Hindu religious art, his tall stature signifies the superior ontological status he enjoys vis-à-vis Shakti, who is in motion. Second, we may recall the symbolism of the union between Shakti and Shiva (as well as of equivalent divinities in the Hindu and Tibetan pantheon) in *viparita maithuna,* namely, the sexual position in which the male sits still and the woman, wrapping her legs around him, undulates her body over him. We may recall at this point that Western "activistic" axioms operated an inversion of the traditional idea according to which the true male principle is characterized by "being." This principle does not act, since it is sovereign and capable of generating action without becoming involved with it. Therefore, everything that is action, dynamism, and development, by virtue of not being self-sufficient, is said to fall under the aegis of the feminine element, nature, or prakriti rather than under the aegis of spirit, atman, or purusha. It is an instance of active immobility versus passive activity. The activist Western world has forgotten these truths, and it is therefore ignorant of the meaning of true virility.

In the period in which Tantrism was developing the doctrine of the metaphysical dyad, the Vedanta system had already been outlined in rather extreme terms by Shankara. I previously mentioned this in the context of a Tantric critique of Vedanta's version of monism. Following the lead of the Upanishads, Shankara upheld in a rigorous way that whatever changes and is differentiated (*kalatraya-sattva*) cannot possibly be real. Considering that our experience of the world is not one of *nirguna-brahman,* namely, of an absolutely pure, impersonal, and solitary purusha, and considering that we live in a qualified, conditioned, and ever-changing world, Shankara concluded, as we have seen, that such a world is nothing but an illusion and a lie. As a result of this explanation, however, the problem is not solved but rather recast in different terms, since we still have to explain the source of this appearance, or fiction, and also how it came to be. Shankara therefore introduces the notion of maya, attributing to it the cause of solitary *nirguna-brahman*'s dimming and of *saguna-brahman*'s arising. The latter is thought of as *brahman*'s manifestation and unfolding in a world of forms and conditioned beings, with Ishvara, the personal, theistic God, at the top. Maya is conceived as something that cannot be explored or grasped; it is enigmatic (*anirvakya*) and beyond imagination. The followers of Vedanta claim that we cannot say that it either is (since maya is not pure being) or is not (since it acts and grows its roots in ordinary experience), nor that it both is and is not. Maya remains a mystery, something that is eminently irrational. Obviously, Shankara denied any relation between *brahman* and maya.

All of this merely identifies, rather than solves, the main difficulty encountered by radical Vedantic monism. The dilemma cannot possibly be solved by leaving the realm of ontology in order to take refuge in the notion of "different perspectives." In ancient Greece Parmenides, who was concerned to safeguard the notion of pure being, formulated the theory of double-sided truth. He opposed the truth characteristic of rigorous thought (*nous*), according to which "only being is," to the truth characteristic of opinion (*doxa*), which accounts for becoming and nature, all the while denying to them ("according to justice") the status of "being." Likewise, Shankara opposes a secular, empirical perspective (*vyavakarthika*) to an absolute one (*paramarthika*). In the latter perspective maya does not exist. This means that achieving the enlightening knowledge that this view aspires to is contingent upon seeing maya disappear as if it were mist or a mirage, at which point one no longer needs to explain it. Maya is but a product of ignorance (*avidya*), a projection of ignorance on the eternal and immutable being.

Yet even now the difficulty remains unsolved, since we must ask how, generally speaking, ignorance and relative perspectives arise. We could find a solution if we were operating in the context of a creation theology typical of religions such as Christianity and Islam. Since theistic religions postulate the existence of created beings (who are somehow separated from God, who is their principle, and therefore are not to be identified with Him), we could attribute to them the relative perspective that arises as a consequence of maya. Unfortunately, in Vedantic monism there is no place for such a notion. Its cardinal tenet is "*brahman* has no equals," namely, there is nothing outside of it, not even created beings that are subject to ignorance and to experiencing the world according to the illusion of maya. If we uphold Vedanta's Advaita monism, we are thereby forced to conclude that maya, in its irrational and miragelike nature, could mysteriously arise within *brahman* itself (since nothing exists other than it). This, in turn, would lead us to conclude that *brahman* itself is subject, in some way, to "ignorance." It is the only way out, but by choosing it, the radical Vedantic monism is fatally flawed.

The following are some further Tantric criticisms. In a sense we may say that the world is not absolutely "real" and that maya, its source, is not totally unreal. A dream may be said to be unreal, but not the power that generates it. If maya is unreal, whence comes samsara, namely, the finite and ever-changing world? Somebody said: "If maya is unreal, samsara becomes real." This means that the unreality and contingency of phenomena and of becoming (samsara) may be upheld only if it can be successfully demonstrated that they do not exist in and by themselves, but that they rather have their source and reason of being in a higher power. If one denies the existence of that power, in no way may the contingency and unreality of samsara be maintained. In such a case, samsara must be thought of as an external and autonomous reality, limiting and altering the supreme principle. According to the Tantras, the only solution to the problem consists in relating maya to a power, or shakti. As an alternative to Vedanta's mysterious maya, the Tantras speak of *maya-shakti,* which is a manifestation of the supreme Shakti or Parashakti. They even appeal to an alternative meaning of *maya,* namely "magic" (*maya yoga* refers to a particular kind of yoga pursuing magical purposes). In this context the term designates a creative art producing real, effective results rather than the art creating tricks proper of illusionists and magicians. Once maya is reduced to *maya-shakti,* there is no further need to deny empirical reality and to consider everything as an illusion.

In her freedom, and in virtue of being "playful," Shakti produces the world of samsara and displays herself in it. Thus the unity of the supreme principle is preserved. It may rightfully be stated that:

> To form a concept of the Godhead that one worships, the idea of Shakti, or power, is for the devotee a surer guide than the nebulous idea of atman [spirit]. It is very hard for those who have no faith in Shakti to trace the "one without a second" through the physical to the spiritual plane of existence, there being no appreciable link to chain the planes together. But a worshiper of Shakti need contend with no such difficulty. In all planes of existence he finds the one power all-pervading. It is therefore laid down in the Tantras: "O Devi! without a knowledge of Shakti, mukti [liberation] is mere mockery!"[13]

Again, it is not a matter of affirming or denying that various things are "unreal." One should rather ask: "To what degree can you make a single blade of grass 'unreal' (that is, not existing in itself, which implies a power over it)?" Whatever exists does not cease to exist at one's whim or thought. The power of action would dissuade anybody from pursuing such fancies:

> Until *brahman* is perceived to be everywhere, and until the chains of the laws of nature are broken and the distinction between the I and the not-I is abolished, the particular living being [jiva] will

doubt this dualistic universe and call it a lie, a dream, and so on. Eventually, the efficiency of karma, namely, the power of action, will force the jiva to believe in it, against his or her will.[14]

Speculative Tantrism, which does not share creationist perspectives, developed a metaphysics suitable for the *sadhaka*, one who is committed to the path of spiritual realization. This metaphysics overcomes both sankhya's dualism of purusha and prakriti as well as the dualism between *brahman* and maya that Vedanta unsuccessfully attempts to eliminate. Dualism is substituted, in this context, with a dyad typical of every free manifestation. Thus we may talk about an "immanent transcendence," corresponding to Shiva, or better, to the Shiva form of the supreme principle. All the powers found in reality have their roots in him, who is both their *culmen et fons*. Shiva is called the "naked one" (*digambaram*, namely, free of determinations) and at the same time "he whose body fills the entire universe." Shiva is portrayed, in a symbolism closely related to Tantric ethics, as one who, while immersed in the vortex of passions, remains free and in control of them. He is the master of eroticism, yet he remains free of lust. Although he always becomes associated with various forms, energies, and powers, he is nevertheless eternally free, invulnerable, and attributeless. The elements that in Shakti's cosmic play appear to be differentiated still do not affect the immanent unity of her Shiva form. Even what is finite and unconscious derives from consciousness, as the byproduct of *maya-shakti*, which is not unconscious in itself. It is important to notice that finitude no longer constitutes a problem whenever it is related to a power determining it.

This context may be further clarified when we consider the meaning assumed by Shakti's manifestation and the "movements" through which she displays herself. While a particular power may be focused on any object, the supreme Shakti has only herself to display, since outside of her, by definition, nothing else exists. In a Tantra it is written: "You are your own birth place; in and for yourself you have become manifested."

This manifestation still implies a "proceeding from" (*prasarati*), a centrifugal movement "coming out from" a state of static stability and "self-projecting." It corresponds to the first movement originated in the feminine substance by the fertilizing action of the motionless Shiva, or purusha. Incidentally, it is analogous to what, in Aristotelian metaphysics, is responsible for awakening the formless power of "nature." The texts refer to an "inwardly cognitive state" (*bahir-mukha*) and also consider phenomena to be Shakti's bursting forth and projecting herself outward, under the influence of a desire or elementary yearning, or of a cosmogonic Eros aimed at creating an object in which to find delight. This phase is called *pravritti-marga*, "the way of determinations," of "finite forms" (*vritti*), which are generated and assimilated by Shakti. In this "descending" phase, Shakti's role is one of negation, since the manifested forms are just partial possibilities of the unmanifested principle resting in itself. It is also said that *maya-shakti* is a "measuring power," since it creates determinations or delimitations corresponding to various beings and to various forms of existence. Ignorance, or avidya, is inherent to power, since it is an "outwardly cognitive state," contemplating something other than itself, which is proper to the yearning and identifying movement of the objectification process.

That process eventually comes to an end. After a descending phase of the manifestation comes an ascending one: thus the circle is complete. The power must eventually recognize itself in everything that is differentiated, turned into an object, an "other," by *maya-shakti*. The process must also be consummated in a possession, since the Shaivistic element must prevail again over the purely Shaktic element and bring it back to itself with all of its productions. Following the centrifugal movement comes a centripetal one; that is, an inner detachment ensues the "outwardly cognitive state," which was characterized by a passionate attachment to those objects produced by *maya-shakti*'s magic (the so-called *nivritti-marga* as opposed to *pravritti-marga*). In the first phase Shakti prevailed over Shiva and almost absorbed him into her own nature. Now it is the other way around. Shiva takes control of Shakti and makes her subject to himself, until an absolute, transparent unity is achieved.

The Hindu Tantras of the Northern School (Kashmir) conveyed this notion through these words: "Shakti is like a pure mirror through which Shiva experiences himself."[15] This resembles Hegel's notion of "absolute spirit," which first exists "in itself," then becomes an object unto itself, and eventually comes to recognize itself in objective forms that exist "in and for itself." This also reminds us of analogous schemata found in Western idealist philosophies, especially when we consider that a commentary on the text previously referred to speaks of the I or "I-ness" in a transcendental sense, or as the essence of the highest experience of Shakti one could possibly achieve.

The same idea is expressed through a conventional analysis of the word for "I," *aham*. The first letter in the Sanskrit alphabet, *a*, represents Shakti. The last letter, *ha*, represents Shiva. The formula of the manifestation is not just *a* or *ha*, but rather *a* + *ha*, *aham*, which is "I" according to the abovementioned meaning of active self-identification, mediated by Shakti, as if through a mirror. The "I-ness" is therefore the supreme word, which includes all the phenomena and the entire universe, which in the doctrine of mantras (on *mantra-shastra*, see Chapter VIII) is symbolized by the letters between *a* and *ha*.[16] Likewise, in Tibetan Buddhism the various powers of the manifestation are ascribed to various parts of the sacred syllable AUM, which in Tibetan too means "I." This is the meaning of the cosmic act of Parashakti, in which a whole world of forms and of finite beings is displayed. A movement ensues in which "duality is dissolved into unity, only to unfold again in the dualistic play." In this movement "*brahman*, which is perfect consciousness [we are dealing here with the Tantric version of the active *brahman*], generates the world in the form of maya consisting of qualities [gunas], and then takes the part of a particular living being [jiva] in order to fulfill its cosmic play."[17] The same principle that achieves the supreme experience of the "inwardly cognitive state" experiences the world as samsara through an "outwardly cognitive state."

In regard to the various ages in which the manifestation took place, a relationship is established between them and the doctrine of the two ways (Right Hand versus Left Hand) in the following terms. The creative and productive aspect of the cosmic process is signified by the right hand, by the color white, and by the two goddesses Uma and Gauri (in whom Shakti appears as Prakashatmika, "she who is light and manifestation"). The second aspect, that of conversion and return (*exitus, reditus*), is signified by the left hand, by the color black, and by the dark, destructive goddesses Durga and Kali. Thus according to the Mahakala-Tantra, when the left and right hands are in equilibrium we experience samsara, but when the left hand prevails, we find liberation.

A further interpretation of Kali's role is found in popular iconography. There Kali appears black and naked, wearing only a necklace of severed heads. Under this aspect the goddess is Shiva's shakti, namely, his power of active transcendence. The color black represents transcendence over any manifested and visible thing. According to a well-received etymology of the word, her name is Kali, since she devours time, "becoming," and progress, which constitute the law of samsaric existence. Her nakedness symbolizes her being free of forms. The fifty heads she wears around her neck (which in popular mythology belong to slain demons) are made to correspond to the fifty letters of the Sanskrit alphabet, which in turn symbolize the various cosmic powers presiding over the manifestation (*matrika*, which Greek speculation identified as *logoi spermatikoi*). The heads allude to those powers because they are removed from their elementary nature, proper to the descending phase. Therefore, if the role of *maya-shakti*'s power in the Tantras is one of negation, then Kali's role, in the aspect so far considered, may be said to be "a negation of the negation." Here we begin to witness the self-destructive and self-transcending orientation of a power that in Tantrism plays a considerable role, especially in the context of Left Hand practices and rituals.

"To destroy" and "to transcend" should be seen mainly in terms of (1) going beyond manifested and conditioned forms, and (2) getting rid of the habit of identifying oneself with external forms, whether human or cosmic. The "destruction" considered here concerns the elements of "desire" and of "enslaving fascination with the self." It is considered a matter of secondary importance if, at an individual or social level, this attitude may eventually require severing relationships and personal attachments. When we talk about the process of destruction at work in the multiform world of nature, we should not confuse it with Kali's attributes, since they serve the transcendental purpose of leading "upward" and beyond (this, incidentally, is the Latin etymology of the word *transcendence*). That is why in a Tantric hymn Kali is presented under that particular Shaktic form in which she picks up what preceded her. In this context, the term employed to describe her action is *vikvasamghera*. In it, Shiva's power, or shakti, is clearly manifested.

Traditional Hindu cosmology knew the theory of the emanation and reabsorption (pralaya) of the worlds, which obey cyclical laws. Such a theory should not be confused with what was previously discussed. It is inappropriate to speak of two ages, times, or phases, if those terms are interpreted in a temporal sense, as if they were consecutive stages in a temporal series. In this second age, we still do not find an elimination or disintegration of the current order. What we find is only a change of polarity and an experience of being as "formless yet endowed with every form"[18] and as "it appears at the same time, with forms and without forms" (*ruparupaprakasa*), which is what Tantrasara claims. Under the aegis of Shakti, who is now reduced to her principle, and of the implementation of that principle, "the world and samsara remain and become the true place where liberation may take place" (according to the Kularnava-Tantra's formulation). In this fashion, Tantrism agrees with that peculiar truth found in Mahayana Buddhism according to which nirvana and samsara are identical and coextensive. This truth will also find expression in the Zen experience of satori.

It is necessary at this time to add a couple of references taken from the Upanishadic tradition, in the hope that they will clarify what I have expounded so far.

Let us adopt as a reference point the atman, or spiritual Self. The Upanishads mention four possible states of the Self in regard to the manifestation. In the first, which is that of consciousness experienced during wakefulness, the world appears under the form of exteriority. In the second, it is perceived under the species of productive shaktis (*tajasa*). Their experience is possible only if one elevates the Self, still operating at a level of consciousness, to a superconscious dimension that in ordinary people's lives corresponds to the chaotic life of dreams. In the third stage, *prajna*, the world of these energies is seen as one; it is perceived in the function of its unity, and personified by Ishvara on the religious plane. One arrives at such a stage when the ego plunges into that ultimate depth which ordinary people experience as dreamless sleep. The law of cause and effect applies only during the first two stages. In the third stage there are only principles in the form of pure causes. Finally, a fourth stage is contemplated, called *turiya*. We say "fourth" in an improper manner, since it follows the other three only from sadhana's and yoga's perspective. By itself, ontologically speaking, this stage resumes and transcends all the previous three. Here is the level of "selfhood" in which the world of manifestations is consumed. When describing the *turiya* stage, the Upanishads say that "it destroys the entire phenomenic world" by "devouring Ishvara as a self-subsistent being."[19]

Another reference is found in the Nrisimha-Uttara-Tapanya-Upanishad. Atman, the one and only, during the first stage is "contained" (*ati*), or embodied, in the material of its experience. This, in a Tantric perspective, corresponds to the function of *maya-shakti*. During the second stage atman exists as Anyatri, "he who affirms": "Atman affirms this world by donating to it its own being; it affirms its own self [as the I of the world] since the world is self-less." There is another expression designating this stage: "it says yes (*aum*) to the whole world," thereby "giving substance to a world that does not have one." The external reality is thus seen as a projection of the spiritual principle's reality, which "affirms" the world. In the third stage experience is simply *anujna*, namely, pure affirmation without a subject or person. This force is then overcome and what follows is the supreme stage, a reference point unto itself called *avikalpa*. Here atman "knows and knows not," which is another way of saying that it does not know according to knowledge that implies an objectification, or "something else," since *knowledge* in this context refers to something "simple," *anubhuti*. "Atman both differs and does not differ from becoming." It is itself "under all the forms of being from which it differs." Hence the following view, which is identical to the "perfect knowledge" (*prajnaparamita*) of Mahayana Buddhism: "Truly there is neither disappearing nor becoming. There is nobody who binds, or who acts, or who needs liberation, or who is liberated."[20]

Aside from these metaphysical insights concerning the nature of the world, the bottom of the descending or the extroverted process is represented by the material objectivity of the world itself, that is, by physical "matter." In matter, the extreme form of "thinking the other" is found in a condensed state. Both the Chandogya-Upanishad and the Gandharva-Tantra speak of the self-hypnotic and magical power whereby an object's thought generates itself and is transformed into it. Consciousness, by thinking "other," namely, a distinct reality, and by following the law of craving, eventually generates "other" and becomes other. Matter therefore is the experience and the symbol of a self-identification carried to its extreme consequences. Only ignorance arising out of desire and self-identification (*maya-shakti* as *kamarupini*), which takes place during the outward phase, makes nature appear to be actual. In the West, Meister Eckhart wrote that even a stone is God, except it does not know it. It is precisely the lack of awareness of being God (avidya) that causes it to be a stone. This is also the case of that particular phase of the manifestation in which Shakti prevails: nature is then perceived not as a self-subsistent reality but rather as a magical/cosmic participation in an idea, in a state of being. We would not perceive nature in these terms if there were in us no *maya-shakti*, which is a similar function at work in our being.

Beyond the limits of nature, the steps of the ascending process—which correspond to degrees of awakening and of knowledge (*vidya*)—are reflected in the hierarchy of beings under the aspect of objectifications and cosmic symbols.

Once these beings overcome the dark passions of matter and

33

break free from the control of their inferior and prehuman nature, they will arise in forms animated by an increasingly conscious and free life. The corresponding limit is the state in which the spirit no longer exists in the form of an object or an "other" (under the species of "otherness"), but rather as it is in itself (*atmasvarupi*). In it, Shakti, instead of being a binding principle, manifests herself as Tara, "she who imparts freedom." Thanks to her, even what seems imperfect and finite now looks perfect and absolute.

From an immanent point of view, the experience in terms of nature and matter of what corresponds, metaphysically speaking, to a series of stages of the one and only spiritual reality, depends on each individual's degree of avidya. It constitutes *maya-shakti's* action in him. However, Shiva, the subject and lord of this function, dwells as a principle in everybody. He is the same supreme power that is experienced in a given aspect of the cosmic play, and he is as he chooses to be.[21] One can only remain passive before *maya-shakti* and be unable to assume it and reduce it to its principle. That is the only reason why the original Shakti cannot be found free and wholesome in every form and aspect of reality, and also why the world is not experienced as release, according to the Kularnava-Tantra's formulation and Mahayana Buddhism's deepest insight.

More specifically, a peculiar encounter or dynamic connection between *maya-shakti* and *shiva-shakti* must be acknowledged in every form and being of the universe. The supreme synthesis may be compared to a flame that, after consuming the matter from which it was kindled, has finally become pure energy or pure act. With respect to that synthesis, every particular finite existence is characterized by a certain inadequacy of the two principles and by different degrees of power. According to Tantric metaphysics, materiality, unconsciousness, conditioned beings, and maya (in the Vedantic sense of the word) all have their roots in these various degrees. In every finite being, the two primordial forms of Parashakti (male and female; Shiva, who is "knowledge," and Shakti, who is "ignorance"; centrifugal and centripetal movement) are found in a different relationship and quantity. According to this point of view, whatever power is to be found in a given being that has not yet become actualized in the form of Shiva is said to be Shakti. Shiva or *shiva-shakti* is instead identified with whatever is unified, transformed, transparent, and luminous. More specifically, matter, body, and soul correspond to the former, the atman element to the latter. In any event, in Tantrism both of them are considered to be simply two different manifestations of the same principle, of the same reality.

Since the union of Shiva and Shakti in both states of existence is not perfect and absolute as in the level reached by the supreme synthesis, the spirit therefore experiences its own power as shakti and as *maya-shakti*, or as something different, even as a phantasm of the external world. The nature of finite beings consists in being dominated by shakti rather than by dominating it. According to the Tantras the difference between Ishvara (God, in theistic Hinduism) or Shiva and the finite living being, jiva, is that despite their being both conjoined to maya and metaphysically the same thing, the former dominates maya, while the latter is dominated by it.[22]

To sum up what has been discussed in this chapter, we may conclude that the Tantras state the intention of reconciling a transcendental truth, namely, monism, or the Upanishadic doctrine of nonduality (Advaita), with the truth proper to every living being's dualistic and concrete experience.[23] This reconciliation is accomplished by thinking of *brahman* as an actual unity of Shiva and Shakti, which are two principles superseding Sankhya's purusha and prakriti. The notion of shakti is what mediates between the I and the not-I, the conditioned and the unconditioned, the conscious spirit and nature, the mind and the body (*physis*), and the will and reality. This notion brings those apparently antithetical principles into a higher transcendental unity, whose implementation is offered to man as a real possibility. In the Kularnava-Tantra (1:110) Parashakti says: "In the world some desire nondualistic, others dualistic knowledge, but those who have known my truth have passed beyond dualism and nondualism."

· IV ·

THE DOCTRINE
OF THE TATTVAS:
THE HUMAN CONDITION

Aside from a general view of the manifestation, speculative Tantrism espouses the doctrine of tattvas, which it borrowed, for the most part, from the Sankhya and Vedanta systems. The term *tattva* has various meanings. In the present context, it may be translated as "principle" or "element." The abstruse doctrine of tattvas deals with the various articulations of the manifestation. I find it necessary to expound this teaching, since Tantrism explains our constitution and experiences in terms of it. The "doctrine of the elements" also plays a key role in practice (sadhana) and in yoga.

On the one hand, ontologically speaking, tattvas are the principles of nature. On the other hand, they are states, or forms, of experience. As far as their unfolding is concerned, I must repeat what has been said about the two great "eons" of the manifestation, namely, that a development in time should be ruled out, since the temporal dimension appears and is established only at a later level of the tattvas' unfolding. The total process includes stages exempt from temporal limitations as well as stages in which time does not have its current meaning:

When we speak of the order of development of the possibilities of manifestation, or of the order in which elements corresponding to the different phases of this development should be enumerated, great care must be taken to specify that such an order implies a purely *logical* succession, signifying, moreover, a real ontological connection, and that there cannot here be any sort of question of a *temporal* succession. In fact, development in time corresponds only to a special condition of existence, one of those which define the domain in which the human state is contained; and there is an indefinite multitude of other modes of development equally possible, and equally included within the universal manifestation.[1]

A modern Tantric *pandita*, P. N. Mukyopadhaya, has compared the tattvas to the image of what appears as a consequence of shifting around various parts of a whole; they coexist in a hierarchy of constantly interchanging functions.

It is worthwhile to emphasize again the relativity of the law of time, which appears only at a given stage of the tattvas' development, mainly because this relativity allows us to solve various problems raised by practical philosophy. For instance, it renders obsolete the question of how a passage of the preexistent Absolute to the realm of finitude may have taken place, since the Absolute does not exist in a spatio-temporal sense. Conversely, it is absurd to locate the Absolute at the end of a temporal sequence of various degrees in the process of realization. At the samsaric level in which it first appears, time is virtually indefinite, without end. Thus Buddhism may claim that no ongoing organic process will ever lead to the end of the world (= liberation). Therefore, Buddhist "realism" is opposed to evolutionist fancies. The Absolute cannot be reached by following a "horizontal" path, but only by following an extratemporal "vertical" path and by escaping the temporal condition characterized by the notions of "before" and "after."

The Tantras of the Northern School (Kashmir) recognize thirty-six tattvas, which are divided in three groups: pure (*shudda-tattva*); pure and impure (*ashudda-shudda-tattva*); and impure (*ashudda-tattva*). Impurity in this context refers to the degree to which something alien, or something of a different nature (*idam*), is found in the corresponding level of each group. According to this distinction, however, even *shudda-tattvas* are somehow impure, since only the supreme synthesis is, properly speaking, absolutely pure. This synthesis cannot be included in the series because it is the foundation and the substance of each tattva. It is called *parasamvid*, a supreme, omniscient power, and it needs to be considered aside from the real tattvas. This synthesis is also designated as a state in which Shakti "enjoys herself" (*svarupavishranti*) and as the I's self-knowledge.

This Shakti "is both immanent in and transcends the thirty-six tattvas and is by herself alone."[2]

From a cosmological point of view, the three groups of tattvas can be compared to the "three worlds" of the Hindu tradition: the world without forms (arupa); the world of pure forms (rupa); and the material world. The worlds correspond to the essential, subtle, and crude states of the manifestation. The groups may also be related to the first three states of atman's existence, which I previously mentioned (in this case the fourth state, turiya, should be seen as parasamvid's complement). From the point of view of the productive shakti, in the Tantras, these groups match the sleep state, dream state, and waking state. Once shakti awakens, the process unfolds until it produces the most distant form of "otherness," consisting in a dualistic opposition between the I and the not-I. At this point, ontologically speaking, the tattvas' development comes to an end. The new series, which is exactly the same as the previous one (this time traveled in reverse), is characterized by the lack of creative productions originating from the demiurgic shakti's desire, and also by states in which otherness and all forms of dualism are gradually overcome. In other words, they are states typical of yogic and of initiatory knowledge, usually encountered beyond the sensory perceptions of wakefulness.

We must now consider the tattvas' unfolding until they reach the level of absolute duality. We will also explore the ascending phase leading to a perfectly developed human condition. Ordinary states of consciousness will be discussed in the following chapters of this book, dealing with practice (sadhana). Practice is not concerned with metaphysical interpretations of reality, but rather with the tasks and the realizations that one can accomplish only by going "countercurrent" and by transforming oneself.

1. The first two tattvas beyond parasamvid are shiva and shakti, which are two distinct principles, but at this level still inseparably connected, whence the symbolism of their sexual union. There is a Tantric saying according to which in every manifestation "there is no shiva without shakti, or shakti without shiva."[3] This is not yet the absolute, transcendent unity of the two (parasamvid) but rather the immanent and dynamic unity of the manifestation. At this level we find the principle of differentiation at work, whereby shiva and shakti are considered separately, as the first two tattvas.

2. After having been fertilized by the shiva principle, Shakti awakens. What ensues is no longer a state in which an immobile being, made of pure light, rests in itself, but rather a state in which

the spirit is the object of perception and enjoyment. At first, Shakti's awakening somehow implies a negation of being, in the sense of an endless sinking into a self-accepting and self-concerned subjectivity. This is the primordial root of concupiscence, and the original cosmic "sensation" that determines the negation alluded to by the Tantric principle "Shakti's function is one of negation." Ancient Greece knew the myth of Narcissus, which the neoplatonic tradition employed in its own version of the metaphysical interpretation of reality. The act of Narcissus staring at his own image may symbolize the departing from the state of being, and the becoming lost in self-observation, self-perception, and self-love (the Sanskrit term *nimesha*, "closing the eyes," is given to Shakti in reference to her self-perception). This is the level of the third tattva, called *sadakya* or *nada*, which means "sound." Here *nada* is defined both as the first movement produced and as the primordial *motus* that originated this dissociation.

3. Therefore, the being that has become the object of knowledge, of desire and, of observation, ceases to be *aham* ("I") and instead becomes *idam* ("this"), in a sort of cosmic fall. This marks the rise of the original element of objectivity, or otherness, as a function of looking "upward." This process, in which Shakti opens her eyes, is referred to as *unmesha*. The corresponding tattva is called *bindu-tattva* and *ishvara-tattva*. On the religious plane, Ishvara, as I previously remarked, corresponds to the God of theism presiding over the manifested world. One may properly speak of *ishvara-tattva* if by the term "other" (*idam*) one refers to the collective possibilities of the manifestation that are encompassed in a larger unity: hence the other term, *bindu*, which literally means "dot." It is a nondimensional dot, encompassing plurality in itself, though in a transcendental way. (*Parabindu* means the "supreme source.") One text says that at the level of this tattva we find a "condensation" (*ghanibhuta*) of power.[4] Here the powers of the manifestation form a unity, which is the image of the I's (*aham*) substance in the form of *idam*, "thisness." Therefore, one could draw a parallel with the chemical notion of precipitation. At this level, the "other" is still totally compenetrated by *aham*, the I, and is subsumed in the transcendent "dot," that is, the dwelling point of Ishvara, who is the Lord of the Manifestation.

4. Duality as such is found in the following level (*sadvidya*), since it constitutes a development of the previous state. Object and subject now face each other and are, so to speak, in full equilibrium (*samanadhikarana*). Hence the title of "pure knowledge" (*shuddha-*

vidya) is sometimes given to this tattva, referring to this transparency, which is still connected to a generic dual principle. The saying "All this [the universe] is nothing but my manifestation" refers to the Ishvaric consciousness, in which the principle of differentiation does not succeed in abolishing identity.

This marks the end of the pure tattvas' series. Next I would like to consider the semipure tattvas, which include *maya-shakti* and the five *kankukas*.

5. Because of *maya-shakti*, differentiation prevails over identity, and the content of experience becomes autonomous. The transparency of universal "pure knowledge," as well as *bindu* (the transcendental dot that includes all the possibilities of the manifestation), is now broken down into the three relatively distinct aspects of knower, known, and knowledge. *Bindu*, through the dyad (maya), becomes a triad, the so-called triple point, *tribindu*. This is the general scheme or archetype of every finite experience.

At this level a split occurs, as in the case of a person standing between two mirrors, whose every movement would be reproduced in two distinct yet perfectly identical images. On the one hand, we have the spiritual series under the aegis of the Shaivist principle. On the other hand, we have the real or material series under the aegis of the Shaktic principle.

Here it is necessary to mention the gunas. We previously learned that in the Sankhya system the gunas are the three powers constituting prakriti and operating in Shakti's productions. In Tantric metaphysics, which does not consider prakriti a self-subsistent principle, the gunas assume a different meaning. They correspond to various modalities of shakti, which come into play once the ongoing process has led one beyond the metaphysical "point," that is, beyond *ishvara-tattva*. The three gunas are called *sattva, rajas,* and *tamas*. *Sattva* comes from the word *sat*, which means "being." The term designates the elements reflecting the stable and luminous nature of being, and it is usually associated with Shiva's nature. *Tamas*, on the contrary, denotes what is fixed in the opposite sense of a stiffening, or of an automatism (e.g., passive staticity, sheer passivity, the force of inertia, weight, mass, a limiting and obscuring power). Tamas presides over every depleted process and over inactive potentialities. *Rajas*, conversely, symbolizes dynamism, becoming, transformation, change, and expansion; it corresponds to what we usually designate as energy, life, or activity. Rajas may also be influenced by the other two principles. On the one hand, when it is influenced by sattva, rajas appears in the guise of an ascending and ever-expanding force, in virtue of which a given form or being becomes and develops. On the other hand, when it is influenced by tamas, rajas appears as the force acting in the processes of alteration, fall, and dissolution. The variety of the world's beings and forms derives from the dynamic and constant interaction of the three gunas, which are constantly undergoing transformation and change. Therefore, in several Hindu doctrines the gunas are adopted as reference points not only by the science of nature (the final result being a qualitative physics similar to that promoted by Aristotle) but also by classifications according to types and characters. Differences among beings are caused by the various ways in which the three gunas relate. Because of the three gunas' interaction the purushic principle appears in the manifested world under various forms.

The state described by the Sankhya system in which there is no longer any becoming, since the gunas are in perfect equilibrium, corresponds to the last of the pure tattvas of Tantric metaphysics. This tattva is found at the level in which the entire manifestation is essentially and transparently subsumed in a great source point, the so-called *parabindu*. The source point, or *bindu*, corresponds to the loss of the gunas' equilibrium, which according to Sankhya originates the development of the world. At the end of the tattvas of this second group, or when maya's splitting function takes effect, it is possible to begin to recognize two parallel manifestations of the gunas in both the spiritual and the material planes of reality. In other words, the gunas play an active role as qualifying powers both in the mental sphere and in the natural world of matter.

6. If *tribindu* and the various appearances of this triad in the order of the manifestation represent the development of what is contained synthetically, essentially, and transparently in the *bindu-tattva*, then likewise, the *kankukas* represent the deployment and the making explicit of what is contained in *maya-shakti*. As we have previously learned, the arising of the experience of *idam*, or of the other, is caused by *maya-shakti*. We also considered that otherness entails finitude, as well as the existence of particular forms, since it exists merely as a part of the whole. Therefore, at this level, what was once the object of a unitary, atemporal, and simultaneous experience now breaks down into a multiplicity, a heterogeneity, and a sequence. The *kankukas* are those transcendental powers presiding over this limited process. *Kankuka* literally means "sheath" or "covering," in reference to the power that veils and hides being. *Kankukas* also refer to the principles of individuation and determi-

nation. They incorporate that particular measuring function, typical of maya, which is responsible for "carving out" and for isolating distinct forms from a spiritually homogeneous reality.

The first *kankuka* is time (*kâla*), understood as the universal form of the elements found in a sequence. Atman, or the purushic/ Shaivist principle, will never fully identify with particular and finite forms proper to a given state of existence. Therefore, atman is led from one experience to another. It eventually creates a surrogate for that totality, which it no longer encompasses at the same time. Atman creates this surrogate in time, or in the course of an endless fragmentation of the finite. Therefore, every state appears to be insufficient, or in need of something else through which its development may be brought to an end. This constitutes the manifestation of the second *kankuka*, called *raga* (literally, "passion" or "attachment"). Once the fullness or wholeness proper to *bindu-tattva* falls short, the finite consciousness is existentially attracted toward different objects, thus originating a temporal succession and the process of becoming. This consciousness is caught in a web of dependencies, which for the most part derive from causality and irreversibility, especially if we consider that every point in time is conditioned by two factors: the previous one, from which it proceeds, and the following one, toward which it orients itself, out of an unconscious yearning for the Absolute. The more this system of interdependent conditionings unfolds, the more complex it becomes. One may refer here to the opinion according to which action (karma) generates ignorance (avidya), which in turn generates more karma, and so on.[5] The point being made is that the state in which being or the other or the very same I, are not "known" generates in turn desire and actions conditioned by desire. Actions performed under the influence of desire tend to confirm this illusory duality, however, and increasingly tie the I to something apparently other than itself. As a result, the I becomes increasingly needy and restless, as it moves further along the temporal series and the process of becoming, all the while experiencing recurring delusions and new needs. This reminds us of a man who is running in the futile attempt to catch his own shadow.

The third *kankuka* is *niyati*, which corresponds to a limitation of autonomy. This limitation in turn is caused by the system of relations deriving from *raga*. The fourth *kankuka* is *kalâ* (not to be confused with the first one, *kâla*), through which the finite condition eventually affects power. Collected and full energy (*sarvakaritrita*) is now transformed into a determinate power, which is defined by a specific existential condition and by a specific body. This takes place on an epistemological level. The omniscient being assumes the form of a "finite knower." Moreover, while at Ishvara's level knowledge is characterized by an objective transparency, at this level it is influenced by various emotive responses, by habitual tendencies (*samskaras*), by what is related to desire, by an *élan vital*, and by a given existential condition. The power that acts in this fashion is called *vidya-kankuka*.[6] At this point, *maya-shakti's* function has been completely fulfilled. Every possible experience is conditioned by such things as peculiarity, multiplicity (in the spatial dimension), time, causality, impulses, and actions deriving from a state of existential deprivation. The difference is that at the level of the semipure tattvas, all of the above limitations have not yet de facto materialized; they are rather considered to be generic, potential conditions for the various forms of finite existence that find their fulfillment only at the level of the impure tattvas.

In the Tantras even impure tattvas are approximately the same as those expounded by Sankhya and by Vedanta. The first of these tattvas is *buddhi*, the principle of every individuation, which is free from every particular form of conditioned existence. At this level individual consciousness appears as a samsaric reflection of a higher consciousness. That is why Sankhya considered buddhi to be the intersection of purushic and prakritic elements.[7] The function of this tattva consists in acting as an intermediate principle between the individual and the superindividual dimensions. Since buddhi is, in itself, on a higher plane than individuation, a continuity between forms and individual states can therefore be established. This continuity, however, cannot be seen from the perspective of those who identify with these states and who are being swept away by the current. The fact that this continuity cannot be seen may even refer, at a certain level, to various manifestations of the I assuming the form of unrelated lives. Let us not forget that the belief in a sequence of existences is the cardinal tenet of the popular theory of reincarnation. With regard to the individual consciousness, which is limited to only one life, buddhi is also called *mahat*, the "great principle." On the level of individual psychology, every decision, deliberation, and determination is determined by it. Buddhi even acts in those volitional and decisive aspects of the inner life.

Ahamkara, or *asmita-tattva*, comes right after buddhi. We have already encountered this term before; as in several other instances, it receives different meanings according to the reference points and planes of existence being adopted. The word *ahamkara* specifically refers to that particular form of "I-ness" which, as in the case of individual consciousness, is characterized by the intake of data of a given experience, both internally and externally. On the one hand, through ahamkara an experience is considered to be "my own" and subjectivized. On the other hand, the I assumes certain determinations to be its own, thus coming to a conclusion that may be thus expressed: "I am this being who is variously determined."[8] This led Patañjali to consider ahamkara and avidya as synonymous, since atman in its essence cannot be localized, being a power over and beyond forms. As in the case of ahamkara, buddhi's determination is concretized and expressed in a given state of existence, which is still conditioned by the ties represented by the notions "ego" and "mine."

The process of individuation is furthermore developed mainly through the third semipure *tattva*, which is *manas*, and then (continues to develop) through the five *tanmatras*. *Manas*, which has the same root as the Latin word *mens*, can somehow be equated with the mind, not as a psychological reality, but rather as an organ and a "power." Thus we may say that manas is the power at work in perceptions, in an individual's reactions, and in the production of images (fantasy, imagination). It differs in two aspects from the modern understanding of mind and thought.

First, manas is other than atman. Mind and thought are not to be confused with the spiritual principle. Manas is conceived as an organ, or as an instrument. According to Sankhya, prakriti (nature), and not purusha, constitutes manas's substance. (This is a far cry from the modern Western glorification and exaltation of thought. Westerners would probably consider the yogic practice of neutralizing or of "killing" the manas to be inconceivable, absurd, and even abhorrent). In turn, manas is the root and the fundamental principle of the senses, and it corresponds more or less to the medieval European philosophical notion of the *sensorium commune*. According to a view expressed in the Bhrihad-Aranyaka-Upanishad, it is through the manas that one is able to see, to hear, to taste, and so on. The senses are manas's articulations, as well as the atman's organs. Manas makes sensory knowledge possible, inasmuch as it is connected to the various powers of sensible reality. These powers are the so-called *tanmatras*, more on which later. As a result of *maya-shakti's* splitting function, they are perceived by the individual as representations or subjective impressions ("names") and as the external reality ("forms").[9] The congruency and correspondence between the two series, which is the fundamental problem giving rise to epistemology, is guaranteed by an essential and preordained unity existing in the manas, albeit at a superindividual and preconscious level.

Second, manas's function, as I said, is not simply psychological. Manas is a power associated with ahamkara and therefore with a certain degree of individuality. This power carves out elements from the totality of the experience by promoting an awareness of some of its areas and sections to the exclusion of others, which are hidden, in that particular being, in the subconscious or in the unconscious. Cosmic experience then becomes, to a large extent, the unconscious or subconscious dimension of the single living being.[10]

Practically speaking, manas's selective action occurs in the context of an experience characterized by the five *paramanus* and *tanmatras*. In order to understand these tattvas, we need to reject the widely accepted notions regarding the process of perceptual and sensory knowledge, according to which perceptions are occasioned by real material objects. The Hindu view diverges from philosophical realism by upholding that there are no such things as matter (in the Western sense of the word) and objective physical realities. A reference is made, instead, to superphysical principles, which come before and are superior to mere subjective sensory perceptions and to what is commonly regarded as physical reality. These principles are known as *tanmatras*, a word related to the idea of measure (*matra*), and which refers to a qualifying, determining power. This determination is applied to sensible qualities, hence reference is made to the *tanmatras* of sound, touch, form, color, taste, and smell. In the objective order of things, namely, in nature, the *tanmatras* are manifested in the five *mahabhutas* ("the great elements"), which are ether, air, fire, water, and earth: hence the transverse correspondence of ether to sound, of air to tangible matter, of fire to form and colored matter, and of earth to smell. The word *matter*, in this context, is only meant analogously, since *matter* in the modern sense of the word is unknown to the aforesaid theory, according to which the only real substratum is shakti, whatever form it may take. The intent is to emphasize that sensory impressions have a definite, real substratum corresponding to their nature, and do not have a mere psychological relevance.

Since the *mahabhutas* belong to the causal plane, they should not be confused with natural elements or with states of physical matter. The *tanmatras*, to which they should be reduced, must rather be conceived as "simplifying elements," that is, as principles at work in those elements that correspond to both shakti's various manifestations and to supersensory forms of experience. The physical elements are mere manifestations and appearances on a particular plane of the *tanmatras* and of the five great elements. This plane corresponds ontologically to the fifth element, earth, which is conceived as a phase of extreme condensation, that is, as a phase of shakti's complete objectivication and externalization. Therefore, the element earth is the principle of everything that appears to the senses in physical and material forms during the waking stage of an individual conscience. Ether, air, fire, and water, which are experienced in the ordinary human contact with nature, are not really the elements carrying such names, but are rather their symbolic and analogical manifestations in the world. The supernatural "great elements" can be experienced. The possibility of a supernatural, extrasensorial perception and of related powers arises only when the manas, in the context of yogic practice, withdraws from the organs of the senses.

For instance, coming to know water means to leave behind its sensory perception and to ascend to a level that is hierarchically superior to the one encountered in the world. As I shall point out, in the doctrine of subtle or occult corporeity this corresponds to the *svadhishthana-chakra*, which is one of the "centers" coming immediately after earth.

In regard to the subsequent organization of a finite existence, one must consider the geminate series of the ten *indriyas*, composed of five cognitive senses *(jnanen-indriyas)* and of five conative senses *(karmenin-indriyas)*. *Indriyas* means "pertaining to Indra." These are powers or faculties related to organs through which the manas, in association with ahamkara, carves out, as I have said, the form and destiny of a given individual existence. The five cognitive *indriyas* are related to the ears, skin (as the general organ of touch), eyes, tongue, and nose. These occur in a progressive order, from hearing (which corresponds to ether) to the sense of smell (which corresponds to earth). The conative *indriyas* are related to the organs responsible for excretion, reproduction, grasping (hands), locomotion, and expression (voice, words, etc.). They are divided into two groups of five: five *mahabhutas* and five *tanmatras*. According to the standard organic-qualitative Hindu worldview, this system is kept together by relationships of correspondence, which are particularly important in the elaboration of a science of subtle reactions, of evocations, and of awakenings.

We may well remember that the unfolding always works from

the inside out, and that the outer, by virtue of leaning on the inner, is conditioned by it. Thus the objects of knowledge depend, metaphysically speaking, on the organs of knowledge. These in turn depend on the "inner organ" (buddhi + ahamkara + manas). The inner organ depends on the spiritual principle, according to the simile "Just as the rim of a chariot wheel is fixed on the spokes, and the spokes are fixed on the hub, even so, these elements of being are fixed on the elements of intelligence, and the elements of intelligence are fixed on the breathing spirit [prana]."[11] The prana in this text is identified with the "intelligential self" (prajnatman). On the empirical plane of separated existences, this identification does not prevent the subject of knowledge from being the "elemental I" (bhuta-atman), that is, the I who is found in the diversified interplay of the gunas and who is, in different degrees of passivity, carried away by its own experiences.[12]

According to the Tantras, this is the whole series of the thirty-six tattvas. Once Shakti arrives at prithivi ("earth"), she stops and becomes fixed. Shakti now stands on the threshold of her own manifestation and, at the same time, identifies with the "other," losing herself in it. The action of manifestation, at this point, is worn out. Shakti becomes kundalini, "wrapped up." She is represented asleep at the center of occult corporeity, which corresponds to earth (prithivi-chakra). She is portrayed as a serpent wound into three coils around the symbolic phallus of Shiva, who is the motionless lord presiding over the manifestation. The three coils symbolize the three gunas. The rest of the serpent represents the forms and the determinations (vikritis) which develop through maya and through the other tattvas. Shakti's infinite potential, which unfolded in the process of manifestation, becomes gathered and lost in itself, in that particular center (chakra) corresponding to the earth.

According to the Tantric perspective, the gunas are responsible for the differentiation of various aspects of nature. In the inorganic world, power is essentially under the sign of tamas. Thus it enjoys a minimal degree of freedom, which eventually is lost in the course of an automatic and mechanical process. Matter in this case represents the objectification of the furthest limit reached by ignorance and, therefore, by the power's passivity as such. In the organic world, tamas's action becomes feebler. In it, "life" already represents a partially liberated Shaktic form, which becomes increasingly free as it ascends along the organic evolutionary ladder. Therefore, the various forms of existence in this world may be considered as the objectification and as the symbol of higher degrees of intelligence (*vidya*). In other words, life is seen as a fire that consumes ignorance. In a living organism, the "other" is gathered to a certain degree into some kind of unity and is perfused by a certain light. Shakti, essentially under the sign of rajas, characterizes outward movement, élan, and dynamism. Eventually, once life is gathered and connected with higher forms of consciousness (e.g., with humankind), then sattva's influence, whose essence is being and pure light, becomes manifested.

Humans are shakti under the double form of conscious, active power (corresponding to what is usually called "spirit") and of unconscious, passive power (corresponding to organic life and the body). The individual's unconscious corresponds to the macrocosm. Through the tamasic form, a finite being experiences the macrocosm and the collective powers hidden in reality. The idea that cosmic forces are locked in the unconscious and in the vital organic elements became the cornerstone of Tantric hatha yoga. These forces constitute each person's occult corporeity. Generally speaking, Tantric and Hindu teachings use the term body (*kaya*) in a broader sense, in reference to those fundamental elements that are presupposed by every individual existence, even though they usually go undetected. Such is the case with a hand, which even though it may be the only visible part of a body, still presupposes an organism as a whole.

In reference to these "bodies" the Tantras follow Sankhya's lead by distinguishing a triple body, comprising the following parts:

1. A "causal" body (*karana-sharira*), which follows the higher tattvas.

2. A "subtle body" (*sukshma-sharira*), which in turn has two aspects. The first aspect is a creation of the mind (the so-called mind-body, *manomaya*, or *vijnanamaya*) in which buddhi, manas, and the five great elements have free play (these are also the immaterial principles that are prior and superior to the various powers of sensory perceptions, which they still condition). The second aspect is a "vital" one (the so-called body of life or of breath, *pranamaya*) that is the substratum of every organic and physiological reality, of various forces, and of vital functions. The mind-body takes up this vital body in the course of samsaric manifestations.[13]

3. A "material" or "dense" body (*sthula-karira*), which is the empirical body, the soma. This body consists of the coming together of the specifications of the five elements (*bhuta*), and it represents

the grossest and most exterior form of the manifestation of a human entity. The material body is sustained by the subtle body, which in turn is sustained by the causal body.

It is relevant at this point to add some other remarks concerning the second body (the subtle body) considered in its vital aspect, because of the important similarities it shares with yoga. This body is an entity that, in respect to the material body, plays the same function that Aristotle attributed to the "entelechy." This notion has lately been picked up by some modern biological theories with a vitalistic orientation. Entelechy is, so to speak, the "life's life," an immaterial and simple reality that unifies the body by penetrating and animating it. It is also at the origin of the body's special form or constitution, of particular relationships, and of the harmony of its various functions. The difference between the Aristotelian entelechy and modern vitalism, on the one hand, and Hindu teachings, on the other hand, is that in the latter, entelechy is not reduced to a mere explicative principle.

Prana, the universal life force, which according to traditional teaching constitutes the subtle body, can also be experienced during the subtle state coinciding with the awakening of one's body. It is said that during this state prana appears luminous and radiant (*tejas*). It is written in an Upanishad: "Life is the breathing spirit [prana]. The breathing spirit, verily, is life."[14]

Even though it is not endowed with breath, as in some crude interpretations of these teachings, prana is connected with the vital "breath" whose five modes of existence are outlined in the hyperphysical Hindu physiology: *prana, apana, vyana, samana,* and *udana.* These are the five *vayus,* a word that can be translated as "currents," since it derives from the root *va,* "to move," and designates the movement of the air masses and of the winds. The doctrine of *vayus* is abstruse for two reasons. First, they are the elements of a supernatural (yogic) experimental science. Second, the texts are not always in agreement as to which of the various definitions of the *vayus* is the correct one. According to the prevalent view, the first *vayu,* which carries the same name of *prana* (the universal life force), has a solar character, and it exercises a compelling and attractive influence on the cosmic milieu engulfing it. This prana assimilates everything that comes out of the cosmic prana. When it is compared to breathing, it represents the inhaling phase.

Apana, which has a terrestrial character, is interpreted by the texts in various ways. It mainly corresponds to the vital energy at work in excretory and ejecting functions (particularly in the emission of semen, in the domain of sexuality). *Vyana*, the "pervading breath," permeates the body, holds it together, and even presides over the metabolism and organic processes such as digestion and blood circulation. *Udana* has an opposite function to the first *vayu*, namely, of exhalation instead of inhalation. *Udana's* unfolding into the cosmic milieu is associated with the functions of speech and pronunciation. It refers to the exhaling of one's last breath at the time of death. It also refers to the ascending current in the *sushumna-nadi* ("most gracious channel") of those who leave behind the human condition in order to experience the active yogic death. In hatha yoga, prana and apana are considered to be antithetical, since the former is oriented upward and the latter downward. *Vyana* attempts to keep these opposites in equilibrium.[15]

Because of its dynamic and lively character, the pranic body enjoys a special relationship with Shakti, since she is, contrary to Shiva, the active principle behind movement and life. The Western Hermetic-alchemical symbolism alludes to this reality when it talks about the "philosophers' woman" or the "occult woman."

The subtle body is usually thought to be the seat of samskara, or *vasana*. The tattvas doctrine, which accounts for the general condition of individual consciences living in certain forms of existence, still does not explain the empirical existence of a given individual conscience, or jiva. We have seen how *manas-tattva* carves out, circumscribes, and organizes a specific experience. Why is this experience being determined instead of another? Why does a certain world, rather than another, come to be known by a jiva? This world must correspond to what the living individual being affirms or desires in its deep, transcendental will to become (which has been shown to be related to the *buddhi-tattva*); hence the broader meaning of *samskara*. The various samskaras correspond to an inner, transcendental prefiguration toward which the discriminating and individuating activity of manas is oriented. In a narrower context, they are subconscious potentialities encountered in the course of life. Some of them have an organic character, others have a psychological character. As one can see, they involve the form and physical makeup of a given body, as well as the temperament, character, and habitual tendencies of a given individual.

We are what we are, even though each of us lives in his or her own world, because a specific group of samskaras is present in each of us rather than a different one. We may encounter this notion even in Western philosophy (Kant, Schopenhauer), where it is spoken of as "intelligible or mnemonic character." The Hindu idea has wider implications, however, since it extends to the biological and subtle domains, as well as to anything that determines the existential situation of a given individual.

What then is then the origin of the samskara(s)? This is a complex question, and it can be answered only by referring to the doctrine of "multiple legacies." Among many popular beliefs of Hinduism, we find an explanation based on the idea of reincarnation, which should be accepted with due caution. It is claimed that samskaras, which are the elements constituting a finite being endowed with body, mind, habitual tendencies, and experience, are the effects and the consequence of previous existences, which are in turn determined by karma.

This does not really solve the problem but merely recasts it in different terms. If in order to explain the samskaras that are at work in the present existence we have to go back to activities exercised in a previous life, the problem merely compounds. In order to explain why those activities took place, we would have to go back, even further, to a previous life, and then to the one before that, and so on, ad infinitum. It is my contention that eventually the series must stop and be explained in terms of an original act of self-determination. What is this act all about? That is an open question. The answer cannot be located in time and in space, since, in these categories, there is no continuity between the various manifestations of a single conscience, or between the multiple existences, as the reincarnation myth upholds. Continuity is to be found only in the subtle, vital (pranic) plane, and in the power of life, which is neither dependent on a single body nor exhausted in it. In a higher degree, it exists in the level of *buddhi-tattva*, the "individuating individual," whose nature consists in shaping reality. One must think that at the highest level of the impure tattvas, an inference takes place in the following terms: pure self-determination, which is a "slice" of higher planes, proceeds from the sphere of pure tattvas and from the causal body, which then translates itself into the act of buddhi.

There is no explanation for this determination, since it takes place in a domain where the supreme reason for acting resides with act itself, where causes are not determined by other causes, and where forms are manifested as stages of what has been called Shakti's "play," *lila*. In these higher planes of existence (*prajina*) there are no antecedent causes and not even samskaras. Samskaras are eventually picked up at a later stage, as a result of the election, coalescence, and appropriation following the merging with the samsaric current. This current includes predetermined forms and various legacies (whether biological or pranic), which refer to previous elements, whether connected or not. In this sense, samskaras actually exist in the subtle body in which the causal body is manifested. They are also responsible for imparting direction both to manas's selective action, through its organs, and to the life that supports, nourishes, and shapes the physical form. Somehow the ancient notions of "demon" and "genie" may be reduced to the body of life informed by a special group of samskaras, which, through buddhi, brings to life the samsaric image of the unmovable Shiva. Therefore, samskaras should not be confused with the real, deeper nucleus of one's personality, which from the level of buddhi on is found outside the conditions for which previous existences took place. This contributes to demythologizing the popular belief in reincarnation, which is not part of esoteric teachings, regardless of what some may think.[16]

So far I have expounded the Tantras' worldview and anthropology. Even though metaphysical speculation plays an important role in these texts, they should not be viewed as philosophical textbooks. The theory found in the Tantras has been developed in view of practical applications, and it plays a major role in *sadhana-shastra*. The theory constitutes the background and the foundation of a system in which action plays a key role. Thus it is said: "All the knowledge acquired by a brilliant mind is useless if one does not obtain the power conferred by sadhana."[17] In the next chapters I will expound the rituals and the techniques of Tantric yoga.

· V ·

PASHU, VIRA, AND DIVYA: THE PATH OF THE LEFT HAND

In the first chapter we learned that Tantrism is a multiform phenomenon. It is crucial to make an initial distinction between the popular versions of Tantrism, which should be considered the survival or, better, the revival of cults and of religious practices found in the pre-Aryan substratum, and the higher forms typical of initiatory and yogic practices. The latter forms, aside from the specific direction imparted to them by Shaktism and Shaivism, are characterized by the pursuit of the highest ideal of Hindu spirituality, which is the "great liberation," or the attempt to free a human being from all kinds of conditioning.

We are not going to pursue the popular versions of Tantrism, since they are the subject matter of ethnology. In them we encounter the cult of Devi, which sometimes is associated with witchcraft and orgies. Later on I will refer to such versions only to point out how they have been incorporated into various types of Tantric sadhana.

It is possible to relate the main expressions of this sadhana to a typology and to the problem of individual qualifications (*adhikaras*). It is a well-accepted opinion that different spiritual paths correspond to different situations. A path that is fit for a particular individual's situation may not be so for another's, and therefore it ought to be discouraged or even interdicted to him. Sir John Woodroffe, talking about experiences that some may consider disturbing, suggested that we should say instead, "This is not good for me."[1]

The abovementioned typology is based on the theory of the three gunas. There are people informed by tamas, by rajas, or by sattva, in whom the respective qualities of each category are predominant. The Tantras make a general distinction between beings belonging to the first type (tamas) and those belonging to the other two types (rajas and sattva), and insist that only the latter two types are fit to engage in sadhana and yoga. A characteristic Tantric notion is that of *pashu*, which is applied to the first category. *Pashu* means "animal" and may designate an animalistic and impulsive individual, who is driven by lower instincts. The word *pashu* comes from the verb *pac*, "to bind." It designates not only those beings who are subject to primitive urges and in whom the material and animal nature predominates, but also those beings who are passively bound by social and moral concerns, and who conform, without possessing "knowledge," to various norms and rituals. Tamas's obtuse and limited nature is amply revealed in such individuals. This, however, does not imply that pashu is necessarily an "evil" thing; according to the common opinion, it is considered a good thing. The Tantras say that during the Kali Yuga, the last age, there exist, mainly though not only, pashu-nature beings. We must acknowledge that such an idea, which was formulated many centuries ago, describes rather accurately the times we live in. A recurrent theme in the Hindu Tantras is the attribution to pashu of all religious and devotional practices. They even consider the Vedachara, the collective Vedic-brahmanic rituals, as something related to pashu, or at best, to the lower grades of the next group, that of the viras.

Vira is a term with the same Latin root *vir*, which does not describe an ordinary man (*homo*), but rather an eminent man. The term denotes a manly and "heroic" nature (*vira* is sometimes used as a substitute for "hero"), which is essentially determined by the rajas guna. Viras in turn have often been divided into many categories. According to the Kularnava-Tantra,[2] there are right-hand viras (Dakshinachara) and left-hand viras (Vamachara). The latter are considered superior to the former, and the text describes them as warriors (*kshatriyas*), to emphasize the virtues of strength, boldness, and indifference toward danger. Next come the siddhas and the kaulas, whose path—Kaulachara—knows no equal. Developing a

Buddhist simile, a text says that "as the footmarks of all animals disappear in the footmark of the elephant, so do all other dharmas disappear in the *kula-dharma*."[3] The word *siddha* denotes perfection and fulfillment; thus it may be considered the equivalent of "adept." The word *kaula*, instead, derives from *kula*. This term, with the ordinary meaning of "great family" or "noble clan," came to designate an organization or an initiatory chain, in which Shakti's real presence is supposed to take place. In this context the Devi is called "the Lady of the *Kula*." Kaulas are those who belong to any such organizations. If viras are characterized mainly by the rajas guna, this quality, by ascending the hierarchical levels we just mentioned, becomes pure and turns into the sattva guna, which characterizes the divya (from *devas*, "gods"), the third element in the tripartite classification of pashu, vira, and divya.[4]

Ascending from lower levels to higher, viras are subject to increasingly fewer limitations and ties. Rites, practices, and traditional cults may be retained, but only according to the distinction between those who have knowledge (*prabuddha*), or those who are aware of their nature and of their superior esoteric, initiatory values, and the common folks (*mudha*). The secret ritual, the so-called *panchatattva*, is the prerogative of the viras. This ritual, which I will discuss in Chapter IX, includes the use of sex and of intoxicating beverages. Nothing is forbidden to the kaula and to those who have achieved the condition of a true *siddha-vira*, since they *are* and they *know*. They are lords of their passions, and they fully identify with Shakti. As the supreme Shakti, or Parashakti, is over and beyond any pair of opposites, likewise the kaula is beyond good and evil, honor and dishonor, merit and sin, and any other value cherished by ordinary people, the so-called pashus. Like Shakti, who is absolutely free, the kaula is called *svecchakari*, which means "one who can do as he or she pleases." Because of his behavior, ordinary people may fear, shun, or condemn a kaula.[5]

There is a significant difference between the two Tantric paths, that of the right hand and that of the left hand (which are both under Shiva's aegis). In the former, the adept always experiences "someone above him," even at the highest level of realization. In the latter, "he becomes the ultimate Sovereign" (*cakravartin* = world ruler).[6] This means that the duality between the integrated person and the dimension of transcendence, or between the human and God, has been overcome. All differentiations and subordinate relationships are rendered obsolete once the Shiva condition is achieved. Quite often, in the Buddhist Tantras, Buddha proclaims the viras' and kaulas' law (dharma) to be "beyond the Vedas" and free from the conditionings to which the pashus are subject. The kaulas are said to be extremely powerful both in granting favors and in striking down their enemies, as well as to be capable of enjoying every sensible object without becoming addicted to it. They act under the different disguises of men who comply with moral and social laws (*shishta*), of men who break those laws (*brashta*), and even of supernatural and incorporeal beings. Again, in the Buddhist Tantras, Buddha paradoxically upholds the relativity of every moral precept, the uselessness of worship, the insignificance of the five precepts of early Buddhism, and even of the triple homage (*triratna*) of Buddhist tradition (to the Buddha, to the law [dharma] and to the monastic community [sangha]), in terms so blunt that at monastic gatherings the bodhisattvas, those who are on their way toward enlightenment, faint, while the tathagatas, the enlightened ones, remain unmoved. Hindu Tantras share a similar perspective: the siddha remains pure and unblemished even while performing actions the mere mention of which would automatically damn anybody else.

Some explanations are in order. First, it is necessary to draw a distinction between an ideal (and those who have truly fulfilled it) and what applies to a specific discipline. Generally speaking, India has overlooked moralism, which conversely has become predominant in the West. In India moral precepts have never been given an absolute, categorical value. Vis-à-vis the spiritual dimension, they are considered simply means to higher goals. Hence the well-known Buddhist simile in which the moral law (*sila*) is compared to a raft that is built in order to cross a river and that is left behind once one arrives at the other bank. Second, and not without relation to what has been said, we find constant mention of the invulnerability of those endowed with transcendent knowledge.

The Manava-Dharmashastra, the oldest Indo-Aryan code, almost flaunts what a Brahman endowed with spiritual knowledge may do without being defiled as a consequence of his actions.[7] Such a knowledge is compared to a fire that in the process of burning consumes every fault (or at least what other people consider a fault). In the Upanishads this theme is reiterated a few times. The lot of those who know *brahman* is not influenced by good or by evil deeds, since these deeds are other than they and have no power over them.[8] In other words, they are over and beyond karma, which is the law of cause and effect. We may add that transcendence of common laws is even encountered in popular versions of

Shaivism, in which Shiva is considered the god or patron saint of those who do not lead a normal existence, and even of outlaws.

The Tantras merely take the coherent doctrine of nonduality (*advaita-vada*) to its logical conclusion. They claim that Vedanta and other speculative schools abound with metaphysical disquisitions concerning nonduality. But how can they be reconciled with the interdictions and restrictions found in them? If *brahman* of sacred tradition (shruti) is truly "one without a second," then what is the sense of distinguishing between good and evil, pure and impure, and between what ought to be done and what should be avoided? This contrast in values exists only for those who are dominated by *maya-shakti,* rather than dominate it. Since there is no other (the other in *brahman* being only the power of manifestation to which it is inseparably joined) on a metaphysical rather than on an ethical plane, there is not one thing that is not pure, good, and right. The doctrine of cosmic play (*lila*), or of Parashakti's freedom, which has nothing above her, and who is not subject to any law, helps to emphasize the point I am trying to make.

The Tantras, while upholding these metaphysical truths, remain true to their pragmatic orientation when dealing with individual practical situations. For all practical purposes, it cannot be ignored that the starting point is given by a conditioned being and that even those who have a vira's qualifications and calling must recognize that liberation from encumbrances and differentiation from pashus represent a goal, a task to be accomplished, rather than the starting point. The doctrine of cosmic play and of Shakti's freedom constitutes the background to all of this. A particular living being, a jiva, is definitely not Parashakti, however, and as long as it remains a finite being, it does not have the freedom to do as it pleases. It may even indulge in antinomianism and have no respect for laws. In this case a jiva will have to endure the consequences of its actions on the existential plane in which it lives and by which it is conditioned. Generally speaking, this conditioning may be related to the Hindu notion of dharma. *Dharma* in this context refers to the nature of a given being. It characterizes it on a samsaric plane and makes it different from other beings. Dharma, which constitutes a being's inner law, is eventually translated into a social norm (a caste's dharma corresponds to the norms regulating its members' conduct). This law may or may not be recognized and followed. From this choice retributive effects arise, according to the law of karma. Karma causes all beings to reap the consequences of their actions, whether they are direct and immediate or indirect and deferred. This is not an extrinsic law, based on moral judgment, but rather an immanent and impersonal law, since an action produces a given result almost mechanically. Therefore, the correlation of dharma and karma defines the conditioned existence of all beings who live in the manifested order of reality.

We should speak of determinism only in a relative sense, since the possibility of acting contrary to or violating dharma (*adharma*) is as real as the consequences that will ensue. It is like a person who ingests a damaging food regardless of the consequences. From an ontological rather than moral point of view, the consequence of *adharma* for any conditioned being usually consists in descending along the hierarchy of beings. In such a being, *adharma* represents the predominance of the chaotic, formless, and purely Shaktic element over the stable, formal element. The popular equivalent of this notion is "going to hell."

The highest Hindu ideal of liberation, moksha, is synonymous with the radical deconditioning of one's being, and thus it implies going beyond dharma and karma. On a social plane, Hinduism did acknowledge one's right to leave dharma and to be excused from obligations to one's caste in order to pursue the Absolute through asceticism and contemplative yoga. I find it necessary to emphasize the absolute nature of the ultimate goal, which somehow eludes most Westerners. The goal consists in transcending and in subordinating to oneself every form of existence, whether divine, human, subhuman, material, or spiritual. It has been suggested that a divine nature is subject to conditionings like every other nature, in the same fashion that a human is bound, be it by a gold or iron chain.[9] We are dealing here with a worldview according to which the world, which is opposed to the formless Absolute, may turn out to be the right key to paradise (*sukhavati*) just as a holy person whose life conforms to dharma may inherit this state of bliss as a consequence of karma. Going from one plane in the heavenly hierarchy to another is not important, since they all are forms of conditioned existence. There is a saying: "Matter and place may vary, but the modality [of a conditioned being] remains the same in both the lord of all gods and in the vilest animal."[10] When dealing with tattvas, we saw how the lord himself, Ishvara or Brahma (i.e., the God of theism), is believed to be a part of the manifestation, even though he represents its peak and boundary. According to a drastic Buddhist saying, which incidentally attributes to Brahma a subordinated position with regard to Buddha,[11] the gods may not experience liberation because they are "dulled" by heavenly pleasures.

According to another point of view, professed by both Patañjali, the great yoga teacher, and by the Tantras, the gods should be considered enemies of the yogin, because as powers presiding over the natural order of things, they attempt to block the path of those who want to become free from it and dominate it.

After this clarification, let us proceed to determine how liberation is experienced by the Tantric siddha and kaula. In this context, antinomy, the destruction of bonds and *adharma* (an action against dharma) are considered means to an end and a discipline to be followed. Generally speaking, such a behavior is destructive, because if it is carried out by an ordinary person (pashu) it would destroy him and cause him to descend along the hierarchy of beings. On the contrary, the adept (vira) imparts to this process an orientation leading him upward, acting in a positive way and freeing him from various bonds. We may then say that the elementary Shaktic nature underlying dharma is activated over and against dharma. Thus *adharma* turns into a ritualistic and transcendental catharsis. It is like unveiling an original reality; or like evoking a Shaktic world in which good and evil, human and divine, high and low no longer have any meaning; or like transcending forms; or like breaking free from the chains; or like experiencing an abyssal depth, which is capable of devouring Ishvara himself. The goal is to experience all of these things without being overwhelmed, to be transformed and to gain access to the Absolute. One of the fundamental principles of Left-Hand Tantrism consists in never becoming separated from the powers of *pravritti-marga*, namely, the descending, Shaktic phase of the manifestation. A kaula should rather assume those powers and bring them to the highest degree of intensity whereby they consume themselves. This is the Tantric teaching of Indrabhuti's *Jnanasiddhi*, which should nevertheless be kept secret and communicated only to initiates, least immeasurable evils should follow: "The yogin obtains liberation through the same actions that should keep in hell any other man for ages unending."[12]

The risk involved is evident. In the Tantras an aspirant is compared to a snake that is made to go up a hollow bamboo. It must ascend and escape at the top, at the peril otherwise of falling down. The texts mention the danger of deviations and the possibility that what is meant as an instrument to reach the goal may malfunction.[13] On the one hand, the Tantras contend that one who has obtained the privilege of being born as a human being and yet does not learn to transcend the human condition is like one who commits suicide. On the other hand, they claim that walking on the viras' and kaulas' path is as difficult as walking on a razor's edge or as riding a wild tiger.[14] The Tantras continuously repeat that the hero's path is filled with dangers and that the pashu, a person with an animal nature—that is, a being who is weak and fettered, unable to rise above his fears—must avoid it at all costs. Thus the ritual of *panchatattva* is kept secret in order to avoid both the dangers inherent in it as well as the misunderstandings and criticisms of outsiders, who are unable to comprehend its deeper meaning. It is therefore necessary to examine oneself, one's nature, capabilities, and vocation, since it is also claimed: "Hard is the great path and few are they who travel it to the end, but greatly guilty is he who, after entering the way of yoga, gives up his journey and turns back."[15] This person is said to be digging his own grave.

It is now evident that adequate preparation and orientation are required. I shall deal with the issue of preparation in Chapter VII, when discussing purification of the will, the symbolism of the Virgin, and the escape from everyday life's nooses (pasha). The main goal of this preparation is to awaken in oneself the Shiva principle and to become firmly rooted in it before evoking the power of elementary shakti. As far as the orientation is concerned, it would be a serious mistake to think that the viras' path is equivalent to that of Nietzsche's superman, or of the hero's path fancied by various individualistic and anarchical theories (e.g., Stirner's). Tantrism does not intend to empower human nature to the highest degree, but rather wishes to cauterize it, thereby consuming the individualistic I and its hubris in the attempt to overcome the human condition.

Before the spread of Tantrism, the Hindu tradition had debated which actions do not bind and which ones do not create karma. A distinction was established between *sakama-karma* and *nishkama-karma*. The former is an action performed out of desire and passion, since the samsaric I is attracted to various objects. The latter is a pure act, and an action performed for its own sake, with sacrificial and ritualistic overtones. Religiously speaking, it is an offering to the Absolute; metaphysically speaking, it is an attempt to reach the unconditioned.[16] In the Bhagavad-Gita the second type of action was facilitated by the lifting of various prohibitions typical of an ascetic ethics and morality, one of which, for instance, was *ahimsa*, the precept of nonviolence. In the Gita the god Krishna incites Arjuna to fight on and to kill even those friends and relatives militating on the enemy's side, declaring that his actions would not generate karma and be considered sinful as long as they were performed in a pure, detached, impersonal way, that is, beyond the ideas of victory and defeat, joy and suffering, good and bad luck, I and Thou.[17] In this text dharma appears to be limiting the warrior's (*kshatriya*'s) way of life and ethical norms. In the end this limitation is not absolute, especially after Krishna, who is the metaphysical foundation and the ultimate goal of the Gita's teachings, reveals to Arjuna the dimension of transcendence and the nature of the Absolute. This Absolute is a power that on the plane of finite beings acts in a destructive fashion, almost as Dionysus Zagreus brings havoc to all things. Therefore, the teaching transmitted to Arjuna culminates with a vision that is characteristic of this dimension of the godhead and that corresponds to the destructive and horrifying attributes of Shiva and of the Tantric Kali.[18] The problem is thus resolved by specifying what kind of action does not generate karma and conditionings, thus bestowing freedom and becoming the path toward total liberation.

The presupposition of these worrisome aspects of the Path of the Left Hand consists in a similar orientation toward transcendence, and in purity of action. We may say that purity also consists in an ascetic action permitting experiences, such as orgies and cruelty, that were forbidden in the strictest forms of penitential and mortifying asceticism. According to a fundamental Tantric principle, while in other philosophical systems yoga (in the general sense of sadhana, the practice leading to overcoming the human condition) and *bhoga* (sheer enjoyment; to be open to every mundane experience) are mutually exclusive, in the kaulas's path they coexist. Such a principle applies to the path as well to the siddha's conduct. A siddha is one who has arrived at the end of the journey; thus he can do anything he wants and go through all kinds of experiences as long as he remains detached and free from his ego's desires. In this situation karma does not take hold of him, since he is beyond both dharma and karma. The difference from an individualistic superman, not to mention from people like the Marquis de Sade, is rather obvious.

According to another Tantric principle, spiritual realization may occur precisely through the obstacle that caused one to stumble. Stumble is an improper term, since it has nothing to do with the religious notion of "fall" or "sin." In the words of Aryadeva: "The world, being subject to passions, may achieve liberation only through them. As copper is transformed into gold through alchemical practices, likewise, those who have gained knowledge use passions as the key to liberation."[19] What is being considered here is an inner change (*ragacharya*) by virtue of which a pure power (shakti) is extracted from what the pashu experiences as passion. This power in turn nourishes the inner flame and leads one to enlightenment (more on which later). In this context intensity acquires a new meaning. Several Tantric Buddhist texts underscore the relativity of all moral precepts, but also declare that passions lose their impure character once they become absolute and once they turn into elementary forces such as fire, water, earth, wind, and so forth. This transformation occurs when they depersonalize the individual (a Hermetic-alchemical expression is "to wash by burning"), thus promoting experiences found outside the conditioned consciousness.

The difference between the two methods is very apparent. Yoga, especially the one influenced by Sankhya, intends to cauterize, so to speak, the source of samsaric "infection." The goal of this yoga is to remove the source of passions and concupiscence, through specific disciplines and techniques, right from the subconscious and preindividual roots, after duly isolating them. Generally speaking, the strategy employed requires nonaction, since any action brought about by karma generates new karma, that is, a further conditioning. The ultimate goal of the Tantric viras is not so different. The method they employ requires not the isolation but rather the evocation and the radical absorption of the shaktic element present in their being. This is done in order to originate a self-consuming process culminating in an ecstatic catharsis.

Both yoga and Tantrism follow a sadhana that excludes anything resembling a repression. In our day and age repression is a rich subject for the so-called depth psychology and for psychoanalysis. In yoga, consciousness is expanded until it sheds light on the darkest recesses of the human psyche. The doctrine of samskara and of *vasana* teaches that the psychological, mental, and emotional states of the ordinary conscious life of the individual (*chittavritti*) are not to be confused with their roots, which, as we have seen, may even have a preindividual and prenatal character, and whose substratum they represent. According to traditional yoga, it is not enough to modify *chittavritti* simply by excluding or by favoring certain inclinations, and by repressing or sublimating certain personal traits or characteristics, as some contemporary moral systems suggest. In fact, according to the doctrine of samskara, once the forms in which a samskara takes root in ordinary wakeful state are removed or eliminated, it does not necessarily follow that the subconscious root itself has been removed. Usually a samskara will remain underground and flourish again, with the aid of favorable circumstances, almost like a fire that only needs new material in order to gain new strength. According to yoga, in order to overcome certain dispositions and spiritual moods, one must reach and inexorably burn down those roots, as if they were sources of infection. If behavioral modifications are to take place, and if these dispositions are to be transformed, one must introduce changes capable of producing a lasting impression on the samskaras, which are the deepest strata of the human psyche.

A different attitude permeates the viras practices and rituals. It is necessary at this point to provide some further explanations concerning the Tantric way of dealing with passions. The idea of the purification of passions acquires in this context a special meaning, namely, that of a passage from the subjective-mental plane to a plane in which powers are reduced to bare essentials (to purify = to strip down). Those who follow this path and the disciplines associated with it eventually come to realize, through a direct experience, that passions, emotions, and impulses are only mitigated, variously conditioned manifestations and faint echoes of powers. What has been said about the theory of the *mahabhuta* concerning the world of nature may be applied in this situation too. The "great elements" exist in and of themselves, beyond their visible manifestations. For instance, the fire of any given flame is only a particular and a contingent apparition caused by certain constant conditions that are mistaken for its cause, namely, fire itself. Thus, once concupiscence, hatred, anger, and sadness are manifested in various individuals because of different circumstances, they can all be identified with corresponding shaktis or beings (*devatas*), in other words, with metasubjective forces. Therefore, one should not say, "I love," "I hate," and so forth, but rather, "A given force is now manifested in me as love, or as hate," etc. The proof of this theory relies both on the compulsiveness of passions and of emotions and on the little power that people can exercise over them, regardless of what people may think.

It is claimed that an immediate experience of this truth may cause a psychological breakdown. Such a breakdown may occur when a person becomes aware of being dominated by supernatural forces acting under the disguise of manifestations taking place in one own's soul (since the soul is merely the instrument of such manifestations). What ensues is a collapse of an illusory world, of the notions of "I" and "mine." A breakdown may also occur when emotions are no longer experienced as subjective reflections but rather as sheer forces. In such an instance they acquire an intensity and simplicity that may result in a serious imbalance in one's personal life. Figuratively speaking, it is as if a diaphragm performing a protective function was suddenly removed.

The Tantric method seeks out such experiences in order to achieve a higher freedom. The secret of its success consists in transforming passivity into activity. Whenever a passion or an impulse manifests itself as a rising surge, one should neither react nor passively endure it, but should rather open up and actively identify with it, taking care to reserve some strength, so as not to be carried away, but to remain in control of the situation. This state is progressively intensified, bringing the roots to the surface. What is taking place is the union of Shiva, represented by the active siddha, with a shakti. One should be careful to prevent shakti from becoming predominant, lest unpleasant forms of obsession should take place, relegating the individual to a "demonic" condition and to a passive instrument of the force that one evoked with the illusion of dominating it. We shall see later on that at a certain level of the secret ritual, the techniques applied to some of its elements are not very different.

If one makes it through this crucial point, and if similar experiences develop in a positive way, the result will be the elimination of one's needs and the demise of the tyranny of various passions and emotions. One then becomes "Lord of Passions," an expression designating much more than just the capability of keeping passions under control, or of totally suppressing them. As "Lord of Passions" one is able to freely dispose of them. According to yogic doctrine, he who "knows" the element (*bija*) of fire does not need ordinary means to start one. Conversely, if all the conditions necessary to cause combustion are present, he can prevent the fire from flaring up. Likewise, he who follows the Tantric path can acquire the power of evoking or suspending at will any passions or emotions, independently from those objects and situations that usually cause them to arise. This may occur with an ease unknown to ordinary people, who are inclined to believe that feelings and passions cannot be controlled and that the only true and authentic feelings are those that are passively experienced rather than those that are consciously induced. In the siddha's case, the passions' shaktis become part of his own being, and part of his own powers. In him, the Tantric principle of the unity of *bhoga* (enjoyment) and yoga (discipline) is actualized. Thus it is clear that the siddha or kaula can do as he pleases, all the while remaining spiritually invulnerable.

Pashu, Vira, and Divya: The Path of the Left Hand

Let us now turn to some practical instructions given to those who follow an analogous discipline. The starting point is a constant, attentive calm. A simile is employed, according to which water, when not stirred, becomes transparent, thus allowing one to see what is or what appears to be at the bottom. A text goes on to say:

> Whatever thoughts, or concepts, or obscuring [or disturbing] passions arise are neither to be abandoned nor allowed to control one; they are to be allowed to arise without one's trying to direct [or shape] them. If one does no more than merely recognize them as soon as they arise and persists in doing so, they will come to be realized [or to dawn] in their true [or void] form through not being abandoned. By that method, all things which may seem to be obstacles to spiritual growth can be made use of as aids on the Path. And, therefore, the method is called "The utilizing of obstacles as aids on the Path."[20]

This is a schematic outline of what should be done in order to experience passions as forces and as shaktis, and not just their psychological and affective dimensions. Their absorption and incorporation into one's being will eventually occur at a later stage.

Until now we have mainly examined the paths available to the vira, a being whose nature is informed by the rajas guna. It is important to recall that such a being may engage not only in experiences related to the secret ritual and in the above mentioned techniques, which lead to a liberation from all conditionings, but also and especially in magical and evocatory rituals. These rituals grant an immediate perception of supernatural forces, beyond the world of exterior forms and natural phenomena. The forces appear under the species of shaktis, since they are forms and manifestations of the supreme Shakti (Parashakti). Thus a magical and highly symbolic view of the world constitutes the foundation of the entire ritualistic system of intermediate Tantric degrees, as well as of other systems. It is also the foundation of most techniques found in yoga, in the strict and spiritual sense of the word. Such, in fact, is the foundation of the theory and practice of mandalas and yantras, which are graphic symbols widely employed by every Tantric school. Mandalas are not conceived as artificial signs, helpful at best to evoke suggestive feelings, but rather as *signaturae rerum:* expressions of the supernatural and objective structures of reality. A magical and symbolic worldview also constitutes the foundation of the doctrine of mantras and *bijas*, the supernatural form-giving forces that are the "soul" and the thaumaturgical principles of the "name of power" and of the "word in action." Again, it is the foundation of asanas and mudras, which are postures and gestures with magical and initiatory overtones. It is through this worldview that a part of the spirit of the early Vedic age, despite all, remains alive in the Tantras. In that age humans did not live as ascetics, struggling with the world and with samsara, but rather as free, uninhibited forces, in the company of various gods and spiritual powers, experiencing forms of enlightenment and supernatural energies, rapt in a state of cosmic and triumphant bliss.

As we have seen, besides those beings who live under the aegis of tamas (the pashus) and of rajas (the viras and the kaulas), there are beings in whom sattva is predominant; these are the divyas, purely spiritual beings (literally, "divine beings"). The Tantras do not mention them often, maybe because in the last age, the Kali Yuga, they are difficult to find. In order to define this third category in the context of Tantrism, we may say that the divya follows mainly an inner path. He does not care about rituals promoting a violent self-transcendence, and not even about magical ritualism. He becomes detached from the dimension of action, like the followers of Sankhya and of early Buddhism. The realm to which he belongs is yoga, the term referring to techniques applied to the hidden forces enclosed in one's organism. In order to clarify the difference between the divya and the vira, we may recall what a Tantric divya had to say: "What need do I have for an outer woman? I have an inner woman within myself." He does not practice the sexual rituals of the viras, who are rejoined with shakti through sexual intercourse with a woman. Rather, he strives to awaken shakti in his own body in order to achieve his goal.

The peculiar characteristic of Tantric yoga lies in the valorization of the body. A classic expression of the Kularvana-Tantra is: "The body is the temple of the god. Jiva is Sadashiva [Shiva in his pure aspect of 'being']. He should give ignorance [avidya] away as if it were an offering, thinking in his heart: 'I am Him.'" In no way is the body to be considered an enemy, and in this context the method of pure intellectual contemplation is not recommended. Tantric schools, both Hindu and Buddhist, perceive the body in metaphysical terms and establish through it analogous magical relationships between the macro- and microcosm. These schools also try to achieve a supreme unity through the correct employment of the body, which must be totally awakened, known, and mastered, in its inner and occult dimension. The hierarchy of the body's elements and powers is believed to mark different stages on the way to the supreme goal. According to an Upanishadic saying, "Every god is enclosed here, in the body." We do not find here a contempt for the body, but rather its employment in the exploration of the secrets and of the powers that it contains.

A further distinctive trait of Tantric yoga consists in a specific form of hatha yoga, called kundalini yoga, in which the acting principle is Shakti, who is present in the human organism. The key to a successful awakening and union with Shakti is to be found inside the human body: "Kundalini is the mainstay of all yoga practices."[21] This characterizes Tantric yoga over and against the yoga of knowledge, jñana yoga, or dhyana yoga. In the latter the body plays a subordinate role; it is valued only in the asanas, which are body postures facilitating meditation, and in the practice of pranayama, the control and regulation of breathing. Outside Tantrism, hatha yoga was and still is conceived as a body of techniques aimed at maintaining a healthy and strong organism. These techniques have a hygienic and therapeutic value, but no higher meaning, so it is proper to speak of "physical yoga." Hatha yoga has been and still is considered, at best, a preliminary or auxiliary phase in relation to the yoga of knowledge. That is because the prerequisites of the latter yoga are a perfect condition of the body and the absence of any disorder and of any organic imbalance that might interfere with the development of the spiritual process. By itself hatha yoga has no deeper value than any other gymnastic exercise. It is indicative of the intellectual level of most Westerners that yoga has enjoyed in these days a widespread popularity, both in the United States and in Europe, essentially under its trivial and ordinary physical aspects, with the exception of otherwise insignificant occultist fads.

In Tantrism, on the contrary, hatha yoga enjoys a different dignity, meaning, and role. As I have said, it becomes the yoga through which it is possible to shatter the ordinary level of consciousness, as well as to decondition one's being and to achieve transcendence. All this happens through a basic power in which both the mind and the vital strength of every individual are rooted. This power is called *kundalini-shakti*, which is Shakti's primordial and immanent "presence" in humans. Thus it becomes an integral and inseparable part of an authentic raja yoga, of the "royal yoga" in the nobler meaning of the word, which reminds us of an analogous designation used by one of the main European initiatory-esoteric currents, the Hermetic-alchemical *ars regia*. The term *hatha*, which implies the idea of violence, may establish a connection between royal yoga and the way proper to viras and kaulas.

Some Tantric orders are inclined to believe that there is a substantial difference between hatha yoga and other forms of yoga, not only in the method employed, but also as far as the general result is concerned. More specifically, hatha yoga is believed to grant an exceptional power over one's body. Not only it is said to produce *jivanmukti*, absolute liberation before the separation from the body following death, but also it is believed to grant the power to subdue the laws regulating organic decay, aging, and even death; to prolong beyond normal limits the span of human life; to preserve all psycho-physical energies; and to have control over one's own life and death, owing to the real capability of committing suicide through an act of the will. The expression used here is "to put an end to the body's life without employing physical means." We shall deal later on with this power when discussing the exceptional siddhis that integrate the human will on the path of Tantric hatha yoga.[22]

Naturally, the chief problem associated with hatha yoga is that of establishing contact with those secret forces in the body constituting the so-called occult corporeity. This is so because the vast majority of organic processes take place automatically. They also elude ordinary consciousness and are taken up again in the unconscious, both in their physical procedures and in their spiritual counterparts. Perhaps the designation of divya, as applied to those people commonly associated with yoga, refers not only to a spiritual disposition but also to an existential condition. We are dealing here with a human type in whom the awareness of subtle forces at work in the organism has not yet been atrophied, as has happened in the course of time to most people. The type being alluded to is one for whom the doors of "occult corporeity" are not entirely barred, or better, one who is still capable of removing the barriers blocking access to it (more on this later).

In order to avoid misunderstandings it is important to underline that the opposition between hatha yoga and jnana yoga is not such that the former can be practiced without recourse to mental/contemplative disciplines, and without disciplines that are supposed to strengthen the will. Such disciplines are the presupposition of every type of yoga. Tantric yoga is indebted to Patañjali's yoga for several of its techniques, since without the mental power of intense concentration, as it is described in the Yoga-Sutras, it is not possible to remove the limits of ordinary sense perception and to walk along the path. What is required of the vira in the Rudra-yamala is obviously required of the yogin too, namely, to be pure (*shuchi*), capable of proper discrimination (*viveka*), absolutely free from the inclinations typical of pashus, and capable of self-mastery regarding pleasure, pain, anger, and other passions. In the following chapter we shall focus on this preliminary work as well as on other aspects of some required qualifications.

• VI •

ASSUMPTIONS
BEHIND PRACTICE
AND THE MEANS EMPLOYED
The Experience of the Subtle
Body: The Bodily Postures

The overall Hindu view concerning the practice of authentic yoga may be summarized with these words: "Very few are qualified for yoga, and even fewer are those who succeed in it." That view, incidentally, should be kept in mind by those who are interested in the discipline at a higher level and are truly attracted to the spiritual horizons that yoga discloses. There seems to be a contrast, however, between the existential situation of single individuals and the metaphysical and general premises of nondualism. According to nondualism (monism), as well as to the theory advocated by the Upanishads, the dimension of transcendence, and of *atma*, is located within the human being.

During the Middle Ages, Albertus Magnus, in reference to the efficacy of the rites employed for the achievement of the *opus magnus*, claimed that "one has to be predestined to this." Several other authors in the initiatory field have expressed their views in more or less the same terms. In some popular Indian expositions the same idea has been expressed by saying that the person who can really succeed in yoga must be endowed with privileged qualities, which have been acquired, through strenuous efforts, in previous lives. Since I have already remarked that the doctrine of reincarnation, from a metaphysical point of view, is totally groundless, we must conclude that these popular expositions merely convey the same idea and emphasize the need for a privileged, innate, and natural qualification. In this dimension what really matters are not intellectual fancies or mere wishes, but rather something organic and essential. Agrippa reminds us that "man's self-transcendence is the key to all magical practices and is the arcane, necessary, and secret thing required to engage in such practices."[1] Agrippa's view, I believe, is universally valid. Usually a distinction is made between "natural dignity" (in which, according to Agrippa, even some elements determined by "fate" may play a role) and a dignity acquired through one's efforts, through a specific life-style, and even through "some religious practices." The privileged qualification, which I mentioned before, is even postulated in India, and it corresponds to the former; the process of an individual's self-transcendence corresponds to the latter. Both are related to what may be called "the true meaning of kingship" (rajabhava). In Tantrism, rajabhava corresponds to the presence, or to the memory or to the awakening, of the Shiva principle within oneself. In a commentary to the Samkya-Sutra, Vijnana Bikshu employed the simile of an exiled prince who, after growing up in a foreign country, all the while unsuspecting of his noble origins, suddenly becomes aware, and eventually certain, of being a king. The ritual of mandalas (graphic representations of various parts of the universe and of the forces at work in them) ends with the enthronement of their authors, who are given, in the center of these mandalas, a royal insignia.[2] We may recall that the vajra, or dorje, which is employed in Tantric Buddhist and Tibetan ceremonies, signifies a scepter—again, a royal symbol.

Three qualities are considered by classic yoga as well as by the Tantras: shraddha, virya, and vairagya. The latter, in this context, is the attitude of detachment, indifference, or contempt toward anything related to a narrow-minded, conditioned, impulsive, and disorganized life-style. By adopting such an attitude, one establishes a certain distance between himself and the world, thus focusing on one's inner majesty. The highest form of vairagya consists in the discrimination between the "real" and the "unreal" (the "ephemeral") and in the radical shift from one's identification with the "unreal" to identification with the "real." That distinction is inspired by Sankhya: reality, immutability, and impassibility are synonyms, as well as the characteristics of the purushic nature, which is sovereign and "spectator." Shraddha is faith, in the positive sense of the term; it is understood as unshakable certainty, which leaves no room for doubts, wavering, or discouragements. Its counterpart is *virya*, namely, strength in an eminent sense, which is capable of establishing a continuity in one's behavior and actions. The texts say that two factors seriously undermine *virya*: fear and desire (including hope). The term *virya* may have the specific and technical meaning (especially in Buddhism) of a force that does not belong to the samsaric plane and that empowers a person to go "countercurrent." As strange as it may seem, *virya* has been associated with the phallus. This explains why Shaivist ascetics used to wear, as a symbol of their god, a pendant shaped like a phallus, or *linga*. The pendant signified *virya*, or virile strength, in the higher sense of the word. One of the recurrent misunderstandings in the modern history of religions consists in interpreting phallic cults in a priapic sense, that is, with an exclusive reference to physical procreation. These misunderstandings were incurred even in the case of Egyptian and Greco-Roman cemeteries (in which the phallus was often inscribed to represent the power of a hoped-for resurrection of the dead) and temples, in which the phallus was believed to neutralize or to avert "dark" and demonic influences.

Natural and acquired dignity involve a certain degree of inner calm or of natural and regal impassibility. When strength (*virya*) is combined with impassibility, it may become what somebody described as a "cold, magical quality." At a certain level, that quality may even be strengthened by "renunciation." The deeper meaning of various precepts, which are usually understood in a mere moralistic fashion, here becomes apparent. Logically, renunciation is a factor of *virya*, of power, and of magical qualities, since it removes and destroys the human condition characterized by desire. The fundamental theory is that every desire or craving found in ordinary people is caused by a state of deprivation. The reason why people crave and become motivated by passion, greed, or desire to obtain something on which they eventually become dependent is that they feel deprived and in need of something. Obviously one cannot dominate or really possess a thing if, just in virtue of desiring, he becomes dependent on it and passive, in the face of the appeal it exercises on him. When one "renounces," or does not crave, or does not seek, the relationship between subject and object is turned around; what ensues is a state of self-sufficiency, wholeness, and independence from things. At that time, it is said, rather than the subject going to the object, it is the object that is attracted to the subject. The object is drawn to the subject as if the latter were its "male" principle, or better, a stable, impassive, and sovereign

72

principle, possessing a magically attractive power.³ Thus each re-nunciation—as long as it is issued from an inner disposition—puts a great power at one's disposal. The occult force that derives from it is called *ojas*. Renunciation is also needed in order to acquire the power to possess an object or to benefit from something without being bound by it. This is, as we may recall, the Tantric notion of enjoyment (*bhoga*), which does not impair one's inner being, and which discloses richer perspectives than those advocated by the arid Stoic ethics and by any religious asceticism. Some texts men-tion certain Shaktis, often personified as goddesses (*yoginis* or *dakinis*), that are irresistibly drawn to the merit generated by the renunciation, and that eventually join those who have practiced it. In principle, a Shakti does not offer herself to those who yearn for her, but rather comes, of her own will, to those who embody her spouse Shiva's calm and stable nature.

I do not wish to dwell further on this topic, since I will discuss later the specific disciplines affecting the will. For now, I simply want to clarify the main aspects of what constitutes a "natural" and an "acquired" dignity. This distinction does not lie outside the dimension called "initiation," which corresponds to the "religious art" that Agrippa believed could bestow the dignity required to perform magical operations.

The monist premises of Hindu metaphysics have underlined the decadence that has affected every domain of life, especially during the dark age, the Kali Yuga. As we all know, in the Chris-tian West it has been claimed that "grace" and enlightenment bestowed by God are the conditions required for "salvation" and for an authentically spiritual life, since all creatures have been infected and "paralyzed" by original sin. Initiatory teachings and Oriental metaphysics do not share the view of this dualistic my-thology. Generally speaking, however, they acknowledge the rela-tive transcendence, in regard to the faculties of ordinary men, of the power that is really operative at a supernatural level. Hence the notion of initiation, which is considered as the implant of a new principle and of a superindividual influence, which are manifested in the awakening and in a particular and efficient animation of one's being. In this we may recognize a special application of the Tantric principle according to which "without a Shakti, Shiva is inactive and unable to operate." Shiva here may symbolize the human being, and Shakti, his female complement, may represent the abovementioned influence.

I have dealt at length with particular cases and with exceptions

73

to the rule. Therefore we should not exclude that, in specific circumstances, one may be able, through his own efforts, to obtain the same results and to activate an operating principle that does not belong to the samsaric current. On the contrary, early Buddhism has acknowledged the possibility of an autonomous realization, exemplified first and foremost by its founder, the historical Buddha, who was the prince Siddartha. Considering the progressive materialization of humankind in the course of history, and the consequent development of physical individuality, later forms of Buddhism, especially in the Mahayana tradition, have reaffirmed the concept of initiation (*diksha*) as the usual way to achieve one's integration. Initiation, therefore, is defined as a real transmission of a shakti, and as a power and a guiding light. While Catholicism professes that the apostolic succession and the continuity of grace ensure the sacraments' efficacy, in Hinduism there have been dynasties of spiritual teachers (gurus), who have uninterruptedly transmitted not only the tradition of their own schools but also the nonhuman power (shakti) that is required in order to expound and to activate that tradition. The image that this transmission evokes is that of a flame lighting another; spiritual organizations, called *kulas* within Tantrism, also follow the same principle. The power is often transmitted from the teacher to the novice through words of power (mantras), in which a shakti becomes intimately connected to a word, thus acquiring a vivifying and fertilizing quality; it propitiates a "second birth."[4] The nondualistic premise is reaffirmed, since this is a birth taking place within one's innermost being. Thus it has been suggested that "those who embrace a person who is initiated into the supreme *brahman* are embracing themselves." And during the ritual, the great saying from the Upanishads is whispered: "Thou art that" (*tat tvam asi*), and also: "Think within thyself that I am He and He is I. Free from all attachments [*nir-mana*, literally, devoid of the sense of mineness] and sense of self, go as thou pleasest as moved thereto by thy nature."[5]

When the texts insist on the necessity of seeking the aid of a guru following this "beginning," however, they may contain exaggerations; some contingent circumstances may even play a role. Considering, for instance, that there were no books containing certain teachings, and that some books were difficult to find, the guru was practically the only source available, even for the most exoteric elements of the learning process.[6] Whatever may be found in various teachings that cannot be transmitted through ordinary language or written expositions should not be overlooked. The same goes for the coded and multivalent character of some texts, which involve a hierarchy of interpretative levels. This set of circumstances, too, dictates the need for a spiritual teacher. Finally, we must consider the continuous relations between a teacher and the person being initiated, besides the transmission of a power, which is not just the guru's own Shakti but rather a super-individual shakti, connected to the initiatory circle to which the guru himself belongs. A positive factor in these relations is the assistance provided in the face of dangers and obstacles, which can be foreseen and rightly evaluated only by one who has already had a firsthand experience and who is thus endowed with a high degree of competence.

In any event, apart from the beginning, which may be considered to be like the induction of the embryo of a supernatural power and light, spiritual development is the individual's responsibility. After this power has been completely assimilated and actualized, the development must reach a point where the novice becomes utterly independent from the teacher. Figuratively speaking, it is said that at the peak of fulfillment (siddhi) the disciple "has his own teacher under the feet," and that "the kaula is guru unto himself and nobody is superior to him."

No matter in what way it has been achieved, initiation has the general meaning of a consecration. Some texts suggest not only that initiation influences the efficacy of sadhana and of the "acquired dignity," but also that, if initiation did not occur, sadhana and asceticism might assume an *asura* character, the term *asura* designating a demonic, nondivine being (the Indo-Aryan equivalent of the Titans).

As far as the technical instruments employed during sadhana are concerned, we may here recall the two main ones: the faculty to visualize precisely ("to see through the inner light") and the faculty to focus one's mind through a training similar to that practiced in classical yoga.

VISUALIZATION

The first faculty, visualization, is particularly required for what in Tantric sadhana is related to images and to symbols to be activated. This is the power of imagination, understood as the power to see with the mind's eye any given form, in all its details, neatly, and not less clearly than through physical sight. At its highest level, it is the faculty of merging completely with a form or an image, until

THE YOGA OF POWER

it alone lives in one's inner space. This faculty is to be nourished with an action similar to that exercised by a lens focusing the sun's rays on a spot, in which at the end, a flame is lit. At this level, we may speak of a "living imagination," or of a "magical imagination." The possibility of some yogic or magical feats, which the modern world considers to be fictitious, presupposes a human type in whom this faculty of living imagination has been developed to a degree unknown to most Westerners.[7] A high degree of imagination may still be found among primitive societies and in some uneducated people living in the countryside, as a residue from ancient times (primitive people should be considered the degenerate remnants of an even older humanity). In the case of the average "civilized" Westerner, on the contrary, such a faculty has become greatly atrophied, parallel to the predominance that abstract thought and intellectuality have gained among them. This phenonemenon is related to a structural modification of the peculiar relationship between the sympathetic system and the brain, or better, the deeper strata of the brain.

The forms in which a vivid imagination is habitually found in many people do not concern sadhana because they are passive forms. This is what happens in dreams and in hypnotic phenomena. Any person who dreams automatically demonstrates a possession, at least potentially, of the faculty to imagine and to visualize, although the person cannot activate, use, and direct that faculty at will. The same goes for hypnotic phenomena. In a hypnotic state almost everyone appears to possess, at least in potency, an imagination similar to the living and magical imagination, although it displays itself only when the conscious personality is suspended and when the imagination is activated by another person, namely, the hypnotist.

We should make the same considerations concerning the activation of the imagination by special substances, such as marijuana and hallucinogenic drugs, in the course of a limited time span. These substances merely induce chaotic visions. Only with the aid of particular substances, and with the categorical requirements of a special preparation and of a favorable "personal equation," may the results be different. We shall learn in due time that the secret ritual of the viras includes the use of intoxicating beverages. And again, only at special times and with the obvious motivation of exculpating themselves from the charge of indulging in orgies, the viras claim that the goals that they pursue in the course of various ceremonies are the enlivenment of the imagination and the improvement of the visualization of images, especially those of *devatas*. In these cases, intoxicating beverages play only an auxiliary role. The essential purpose of their ritual use does not bear a relation to the specific problem being here considered, namely, that of the awakening of the imagination when that faculty is absent from the very beginning. This essential purpose consists in the induction of a state that in ancient Greece was known by a term carrying a positive connotation, *mania*. This state was characterized by a "divine enthusiasm" and by a feeling of rapture similar to that experienced in Dionysianism and in the Dionysian use of wine and of sacred orgies for initiatory purposes.

When it is a matter of training and of developing a faculty that is partially present, some methods are indicated, such as recollection. One should first focus on an object located before one's eyes, and then try, after closing the eyes, to see it only with the mind's eye. In a following exercise, after opening the eyes, one should see the object "out there" in space, as if it were a real thing.[8] In all likelihood, many psychiatrists would consider this exercise as a way to induce hallucinations. In so doing, however, they would miss the main point: what are being propitiated through this method are not compulsive and involuntary processes, as in the case of real hallucinations. Usually, the result being sought is exactly the opposite of becoming a victim of one own's imagination.

We may also consider cases such as a sudden enlightenment, for instance, the one experienced, in the case of physical sight, by the surgical removal of cataracts. The cause of such an experience may be the adding up of imponderable factors until they reach a critical breaking point, or even a successful contact with certain supernatural influences, which confer to the phenomenon an initiatory meaning. This is what apparently happened to Gustav Meyrink, the author of interesting novels with initiatory overtones. Meyrink had practiced yogic techniques for a long time without satisfactory results, because he used to think with words, like many other intellectuals, and was unable to see figures, forms, and colors through the mind's eye. Meyrink had given up those techniques when one day, finding himself in a peaceful state of mind before a winter landscape, he had a vision: he saw in the sky a figure in the characteristic crossed-legs posture that is attributed to Buddha. That was for him the sudden, miraculous opening of the mind's eye. He felt like a horse who had started to gallop after sleepily walking along for a long time.

As far as visualizations are concerned, the Tibetan Tantras

distinguish two procedures. The first is the sudden "projection" of the whole image, which is compared to a fish darting out of water. The second is gradual; the image is composed a part at a time, since each part, or each attribute in the case of a personified ritual image, must act almost as if it were added fuel, which intensifies the mental fire.[9]

The importance of the imagination consists in being the necessary instrument, allowing one to move on the subtle plane. Some people, through the intensity of their imagination and their power of concentration on a single image, eventually become removed from physical perceptions and from the sense of their own bodies and come to "see" only through their inner light. To these people it is given to enter in contact with forces that belong to the order of things that includes the "mental body" and the "body of life," as well as things such as "names," "seals," and "elements," which I have mentioned when dealing with the Tantric worldview. The entire cult, in the evocative sense found at the highest levels of Tantrism, consists of animations caused by the power of the magical and living imagination. The same can be said about the bodily postures (asanas) and the ritual gestures (mudras). We may apply here the Tantric principle according to which the human Shiva is almost paralyzed and unable to act, unless he is connected with this Shakti.

A particular application of the power of visualization concerns what in China has been called "to act without acting." For clarity's sake let us refer to our own bodies. As we all know, there are two ways to move the body; one way is direct, through an order transmitted by the brain. The other is indirect, flowing out of a reflex, and is induced by an idea, through the imagination. An example of the latter may be the physiological and mimic rebound caused in a spectator by the sight of a trapeze artist's sudden fall. Another example is the physiological phenomenon of sexual arousal, which may be induced by evoking in one's mind erotic scenes. These examples, as well as many others, testify to an "effortless" aspect of the imagination that controls movement, and that should be distinguished from the muscular-volitive action, which is capable of reaching domains precluded to the latter.

A particular importance is given to the development of this faculty, since it may affect various domains; the faculty of moving or of determining things through an act of the mind, with "images-commands," effortlessly and without recourse to what may be called one's jivalike physical will. A relation may be eventually established with the notion of *vajra*, the "diamond thunderbolt" which Tibetan Buddhism employs in its operating procedures.

Let us now deal with the second fundamental instrument, represented by the capability of unifying and focusing the mind.

UNIFICATION OF THE MIND

It is easier to achieve results through unifying the mind than through visualization. In yoga manuals, Patañjali's included, we find the outline of a corresponding gradual discipline.[10] The starting point is usually represented by five states of mind:

1. Unstable, changing, wavering (*ksipta-chitta*)
2. Inattentive, confused (*mudha*)
3. Occasionally focused (*vikshipta*)
4. Gathered in only one spot (*ekagriya* or *ekagrata*)
5. Completely mastered (*niruddha*)

The first two states are found predominantly in the common person, in the pashu. Rather than thinking, such a person "is thought"; various impressions arise, develop, create patterns, proliferate, and eventually disappear within him in a kaleidoscopic vortex over which he has little or no control, and by which he is carried. A well-known Hindu simile is that of a monkey that is difficult to catch, since it ceaselessly jumps from branch to branch. The third state (*vikshipta*), even though it belongs to ordinary life, is a different case. There are situations in which the mind successfully concentrates and remains alert for a short while, as in the case of watching a theater production, or reading something interesting, or being absorbed in a certain feeling or preoccupation, or trying to solve a problem or to recognize a sound, or remembering something, and so on. This state, too, is not a positive one. Here, in fact, what takes place is a "passive attentiveness," since it is the object itself, or a given interest, that originates the momentary concentration. Anyone will agree with me, simply by trying to concentrate on something that he considers absolutely irrelevant to his life; after a minute or two, he will catch his mind wandering somewhere else.

Only in the fourth state, in which one actively concentrates on one spot (*ekagriya*), does the mind begin to be a useful instrument for yoga and for sadhana in general. This state, however, is not easy to achieve. When the Hindu texts describe *ekagriya* as something that is naturally presupposed in the disciple or in their readers, they should not be misunderstood; one may achieve *ekagriya* only through perseverance and tireless application.

The discipline that is employed consists in reducing to a minimum the role that the first two states play in ordinary life. This is done in order to bring about a stable and continuous self-awareness, as well as a methodical de-identification with the sensations (*vrittis*), and also with the fluctuating and mobile contents of inner and outer experiences. The goal is achieved when the passive and scattered states are removed, and they cease to be habitual states of consciousness; at this point, the obtuse coalescence of the I with mental modifications has finally been overcome. The following are the recommended initial exercises that lead to de-identification.

With a calm mind, leave thoughts to themselves. Witness the sight of various mental associations being formed spontaneously and capriciously, without losing your self-awareness; do not disturb them, but do not let them carry you away. Carefully avoid entertaining or developing any thought that solicits your imagination. It may be useful to reformulate mentally the thoughts that knock at your mind's doors, by saying: "So there! Now I have this thought, and previously I have entertained that thought," and so on. Since, at the beginning, it often happens that the mind wanders off, when that happens, one should not go on. Instead of starting from the very last thought, one should rather attempt to reconstruct the path of the fleeing thoughts that have preceded the last thought, and then start again from the point in which one enjoyed self-awareness.

Some texts refer to this technique as the "shepherd's exercise." One's inner attitude resembles that of a shepherd who leads his flock to the pasture and lets it roam free, without ever losing sight of it. The positive result is achieved—this too is an image found in the texts—when one experiences a feeling similar to the one experienced by a calm person who sits on the bank of a river and watches the water flow by.

The same result is achieved through another method, the so-called cutting-off method. One must remain alert and suppress every thought and mental image, as soon as it surfaces in the mind, just as a quick, clean slash with a sickle easily mows down a blade of grass. Whenever a new thought surfaces, it should be dealt with the same way. After a while, if one successfully persists, he will eventually witness a sort of flight of thoughts and images; this is the "view of the fleeing enemy," which is contingent on the I becoming detached from the contents of its own consciousness. One will thus find himself in the same final condition arrived at in the previous exercise, experiencing the peaceful state of mind of one who sits by a river's bank, watching the water flow by.[11]

These exercises ought to be applied eventually to ordinary situations, which are particularly plagued by associative automatisms. I am referring to mental contents that take form and succeed one another while one is traveling from one place to another, or while eating, getting dressed, and so on. These contents are habitually consumed moment by moment, and the subject is rarely aware of them (the proof is that if one suddenly halts the mental flow, he will hardly remember what he was thinking about just moments ago).

An analogous de-identification is postulated in regard not only to mental modifications but to emotional states as well. The task here is much more difficult. It consists in objectifying and looking at one's own feelings and emotions, as if in a mirror. The path that leads the apprentice, little by little, to the goal does not consist in taking upon oneself the most recent feelings, emotions, or impulses, not even as they occur, but it consists in assuming those past ones, which arose in different circumstances. They are to be regarded with calm and detachment, as if they were somebody else's. This is done by imagining them to arise, develop, and become transformed into another person, for whom we care little. Thus, slowly, one becomes inclined to adopt the same attitude even regarding analogous present states.[12]

At this level, one should experience as natural and normal the following realizations of sadhana: a calm presence unto oneself, the dissociation of the I from *chittavrittis*, and a remarkable reduction of the *ksipta-chitta* and of the *mudha-chitta* states.

This yoga training is the necessary antecedent to the practice of classical yoga, according to the doctrine expounded in Patañjali's Yoga-Sutras and eventually clarified in several commentaries to his work. This yoga is a system in itself; generally speaking, the techniques expounded in it are believed to be sufficient to lead the apprentice to total liberation, at least according to one of its interpretations, which was heavily influenced by Sankhya. When considering the classical phases of mental concentration and of yogic contemplation, I will not put the emphasis on classical yoga's perspectives (the subject matter of this book, after all, is Tantrism) and on their actualization. I believe in fact, that they merely constitute a necessary instrument to sadhana in general; they also happen to

THE YOGA OF POWER

foster the living imagination, which I have already discussed. The power I am going to discuss has been called *samyama,* and it develops through some phases of sadhana that I want to describe briefly. I had mentioned previously that it approximately corresponds to the acquisition of a power that in some European philosophical circles is called "intellectual intuition." This intuition consists in the identification of knowing and being beyond the external, sensible, mental, and phenomenal forms that are encountered in ordinary experiences.

The first phase of the process of realization, *pratyahara,* is the actualization of the mind's de-identification from various impressions and stimuli. The object is to gather the mind in itself, in its substance, through the power of excluding, at will, sensory impressions and mental modifications. The theory behind it is not that one sees through the eye or hears through the ear, but that it is the manas that sees through the eye, hears through the ear, and so on. Thus it is possible for the manas to withdraw from these sensory organs. It withdraws, in the first place, in order to focus the mind on an inner object; second, in order to perceive sensations and feelings in their true nature; and last, in order to achieve a state analogously called "silent."

As far as the second state is concerned, I have already mentioned this power when speaking of the stripping of passions and emotions, which is practiced in the Path of the Left Hand. The term employed in yoga to define mental modifications is *vritti.* The assumption behind this term is that in the course of the habitual identification of the I with its experiences, the subject perceives only weak reflections, while the real source of the corresponding processes is to be found in one's heart. That the Chinese ideogram for "thought" is the same as that for "heart" may or may not be related to this, or may be a faint echo. Something of this sort is also documented in the ancient Egyptian language. When the mind, through pratyahara, withdraws inside itself, it is said that ideas and thoughts may be perceived in a flash of pure energies that are issued from a central part of the body and that strike the brain. After all, this is suggested by the term *vritti,* which does not literally mean "modification," "state," or "form," but rather "whirlwind" or "vortex." Thus, in relation to the abovementioned experience, the Tantric Tibetan texts describe thoughts as meteorites, or as flying arrows, and even as flashes.[13]

As far as the "silent" state pursued by manas is concerned, it is the state in which the spirit calmly rests within itself. We may think of the relationship between the I and thought as being analogous to the relationship between the I and speech. As silence ordinarily consists in refraining from talking and in not activating speech, likewise, one should refrain here from activating thought and keep it still and gathered. The various thoughts that follow one another in ordinary life might be compared to talking instinctively and randomly. In pratyahara, through a calm action, talking chaotically is suspended: one remains silent, experiencing the mind's inner silence. Such a silence usually precedes and follows every session of sadhana.

The second phase of the process of realization, *dharana*, may be considered a development of *ekagriya*. The stasis of the mind gathered in itself is shattered, and the spirit now focuses on only one object, excluding everything else, including sensory impressions, thoughts, and causal mental associations. In order to distinguish dharana from *ekagriya*, which consists in the mind focusing on only one place, it is necessary to relate dharana to the third and following phase of the process of realization, which is called *dhyana*; this third phase has a noetic character and a cognitive penetration of the chosen object. In itself, dharana is sometimes thought of as a process facilitating hypnosis, since it is believed to neutralize thought and to free purely spiritual energy, which is thus enabled to act without being bound to the senses. Thus, Vyana suggests that the places that may be the basis of dharana are the top of the head, the navel, the tip of the nose, the roof of the palate, or even an external object or sound.[14] Obviously, the process of isolating oneself from external impressions, like hypnosis, is just a means to an end. Yoga has absolutely nothing to do with any hypnotic or trancelike state. Yoga, on the contrary, pursues a greater consciousness and a higher than normal clearheadedness.

Another possibility, always within the context of dharana, consists in assuming the same object, image, symbol, or phenomenon chosen for the following phase, or dhyana, as the basis or the support for the neutralization of thoughts. What will ensue is some kind of continuity, and the passage from a merely technical phase to a phase of spiritual realization. One should not attempt, at first, to neutralize those thoughts that are connected to the brain and to one's detachment from external factors. One should rather consider that the total absorption of the I into the object to be disclosed leads automatically to the spirit's release from all bonds.

The third phase of the process of realization, *dhyana*, is the third articulation *(anga)* of classical yoga. It consists in the assimilation and in the actual interiorization of the object that is contemplated. Here, the absolute unity and continuity of the mental current is especially stressed. According to a simile that I have already employed, this current resembles a solar ray, which a lens focuses on the same spot, without interruption, at the right distance, until the object situated in the mind catches fire. This therefore has nothing to do with hypnotic suggestion—which can only be, as I have said, an auxiliary and subordinated tool—but is rather an essentially intellectual and suprarational process. The object must be penetrated in all of its aspects and examined from every possible perspective, letting it say what it is in its essence. One will then be able to perceive it in its unity and in a synthesis that regards its existence as secondary. Another image that may be employed is that of a welding torch aimed at one spot until the metal melts. The metal, in this case, symbolizes what in the object is external, sensible, or perceived by the imagination.

The fourth and last phase is called *samadhi*. If we employ again the simile of the welding torch, samadhi would correspond to the moment in which the fusion takes place. In it, the *idam* element (= otherness) of the object is finally removed. Also, the cognitive act and the object of contemplation cease to be distinct, just as a difference cannot be established between the image of a thing and its essence. We are here projected beyond the sensible world of phenomena, beyond the subjective world of thoughts and of simple imaginations. The element called "form" is eliminated, and what remains is the essence (*artha*) of a thing, or the power (shakti) of a thing, figure, or symbol. What remains is the power of what was placed in the "fire" of the process, which is now revealed to the apprentice, in a direct and eminently objective experience.

The term *samadhi* is used prevalently in the context of jnana yoga. Tantrism, on the other hand, employs more frequently the term *bhava*, which has a technical meaning (otherwise *bhava* may signify "nature," "disposition," or "state"). *Bhava* is said to be the essential organ in Shakti's dimension, since the shakti of everything that appears as "other" is revealed only through it. Without *bhava*, according to the Kauvali-Tantra, it is impossible to acquire a high degree of competence in the kaulas' doctrine. One text declares that whoever is capable of realizing a perfect *bhava* does not need anything else, since he already possesses the organ for the real knowledge of Shakti. It is only natural that such a state may be difficult to understand for those who have never experienced it, one way or another. It is said: "How can the true nature of *bhava* be expressed in words? *Bhava* cannot be described. Words can only indicate the direction in which it is to be found."

There are various degrees in the process of spiritual realization, depending on the object that has been chosen. If the basis consists in an object of sensory experience, in order to arrive at *bhava* it is necessary to go through a double process of abstraction. At first the object, as it is perceived by the senses, is excluded; once every other representation of this object is excluded through pratayahara, what remains is only an image. Once this image is contemplated and animated in one's inner light, this very support, or facsimile, is abolished, in the same way that physical perception was suppressed. The consequence is the arising of some kind of secondary reflection, which is formless and immaterial, and from which *bhava* eventually develops. *Bhava* corresponds to the "formless" or "causal" plane (*arupa, karana*), while the previous reflection, which may be attributed to the phase of dhyana, corresponds to the subtle plane.

When the starting point is not a physical object but an inner object, namely, an image, a feeling, and so forth, such a starting point consists in the neutralization of the outer sensibility; what is left are the two remaining phases.

Commentators on Patañjali's Yoga-Sutras distinguish various degrees of samadhi. The reference point consists in the state in which the object, the concept, or the representation appears radically distinct from its name. The lower form of samadhi (or *bhava's* samadhi) is one in which the concept and its name still subsist, and both of them are conditioned by a specific existence, culture, language, and time period. Thus the real nature of the object is still hidden behind a veil. This nature is grasped in the higher form of samadhi, called *nirvitarka*. In this form the object is stripped of any association with names and with concepts, through an intensification of the intellectual fire, and is also stripped of the same relationship with a specific being's I. Therefore, it is penetrated into the essential nakedness of its own nature (*svarupa*). We may say that, in this context, the magic of maya, in the Vedantic understanding of the word, is shattered. Therefore, the human sight participates in the nature of Shiva's sight; Shiva, with his symbolic frontal ("cyclopic") eye, destroys everything that in the manifestation clothes and covers nescience. A parallel to this notion may be found in the ancient Greek notion of the "Olympian stare," or *nous*, to which the higher reality of the so-called *kosmos noetos* is revealed over and beyond the world of phenomena. The yogic technical term *samyama* is employed to describe the whole process, which includes dharana, dhyana, and samadhi.

If *samyama* is applied to sensible objects, the *bhava* state, in its perfection, may put the apprentice in direct and experimental contact with the transcendental elements and with the principles of the senses and of the sensible objects (*tanmatras* and *mahabhutas*).[15] These contacts correspond either to as many forms of knowledge-enlightenment (prajna) or to perceiving faculties, which are not conditioned by the body's organs.[16] Mention is made of the possibility of seeing without eyes, touching without hands, hearing without ears, arriving without departing, and so on.[17] In the third book of the Yoga-Sutras these various possibilities of *samyama* are described in detail.

It must be acknowledged that the term *samyama* may be used to refer to an extraordinary and enlightening knowledge both of the powers and of the essences that are manifested in the external world, and also of those powers and essences whose manifestation habitually takes place within the realm of feelings and emotions. *Samyama* may also be focused on powers and entities that are found on planes and on existential levels having no immediate correspondence to ordinary human experiences. In this case the basis for the process of disclosure consists in symbols, figures, sounds, and signs, which are described by various esoteric traditions. The magical procedures of Tantric rituals and of hatha yoga are essentially based on this material, which is described in esoteric traditions and which is outlined in a direct teaching.

I hope that my exposition of the articulations of classical yoga has helped the reader to believe in the existence of processes that are properly ordained to the supreme goal and that consist in the liberation of the I and in the deconditioning of one's being (Tantrism follows a different path from that of hatha yoga). Several forms of samadhi must be distinguished. The faculty necessary to make this distinction is attributed to the highest of these forms. This form is not applied to particular objects or goals; it no longer has any "support"; and it is ordained only to the knowledge-realization of *atma*. As far as my research is concerned, I shall focus only on those elements concerning the formation of a working tool; such, in fact, is the power of *samyama* in an elementary and approximate form, since it feeds the mental fire in order to promote the development of an extrasensory perception.

In regard to hatha yoga, one of the first applications of this instrument concerns one's own body. The goal is to gradually acquire a subtle perception of it and of the forces acting in it. One of the misunderstandings that the yoga practiced in the West has generated is to believe in the existence of physical methods leading to spiritual realizations. This is absolutely preposterous; when the Hindu texts speak about the physique, they are actually referring to something very different from what our contemporaries, especially modern Europeans, mean by that term. One of its obvious premises, which does not even need to be enunciated, is that a yoga apprentice's body was, and still is to a greater extent, penetrated by the I, and that it was, or still is, more intimate and disclosed to the I in its subtle dimension. Thus even the physical procedures considered by yoga have implications that are not merely physical.

In any event, exercises promoting an intense concentration are indicated. These exercises focus on functions, organs, or particular areas of the body in order to systematically expand one's consciousness by moving into the organic unconscious. The result is the dematerialization and the shift onto a subtle plane of what is commonly called coenesthesia (the overall sensation of the organism).

Breathing is particularly important in all this, considering the role it plays in almost every form of yoga, especially in kundalini yoga. The effectiveness of the control of breathing (pranayama) presupposes a contact with the subtle dimension; what truly matters in yogic practice, with the exception of exercises found in mere physical yoga, is the breath that is the life force (prana), and not breath in its coarse form (*sthula*). Training consists in lying down, relaxing, and waiting for breath, once completely abandoned to itself, to assume a regular rhythm, "as in a sleeping child." At this time, one should begin to progressively concentrate on one's breathing. According to the texts, the sensation of prana is analogous to that of a diffused light; it may generate the feeling of warmth in the following phase, when this interiorization shifts from the breathing function to the related function of blood circulation.[18] At this phase, one's level of consciousness has already shifted. We shall learn how in yoga, one's breath is considered a vehicle to go from ordinary waking consciousness to deeper forms of consciousness, which are kept hidden from common people by the dreaming state and by various levels of sleep.

This consciousness is thought to be the way to enter within one's body, to experience that life which is usually beyond and outside one's reach. This descent takes place in a natural way every night when we fall asleep, or better, when we yield to sleep. But ordinary consciousness is not able to keep up with this change of state and of level; it is barred from entering it, as if it was guarded by a stern angel standing by the Tree of Life.[19] Only when the power of abstraction and of contraction has developed beyond a certain level may this situation be partially modified. Some forms of meditation are suggested as a starting point. I will just mention one of them.

At night, before going to sleep, one should visualize a sun that gradually rises above the horizon until it reaches all of its splendor in the middle of a fully lit sky. The image should be vivid and filled with the feeling of one's being elevated, opening up, and becoming illuminated. One should also think that such a mental image corresponds to what will really take place in the deep of the night, when that midnight sun, known also to ancient Western mysteries, shines with all its radiance. The zenith of this sun should be conceived as the point in which one's identification with the light and with a sense of liberation has become perfect. One should then try to fall asleep right away, before other images or other thoughts may crop up in the mind. Early in the morning, once completely awake, one should image the midnight sun and make it descend from its zenith to its setting (which in this inversion corresponds to the rising of the sun). One should also feel that the light that fades away when the physical daily light begins to shine, lights up within one's self and keeps shining during one's waking state. In this fashion, one generates a sense of a light opposite to that which shines in the natural world and which allows the physical eyes to see.

Such a practice is believed to enhance the subtle perception of one own's body and life as well as an initial integration of consciousness in a state that corresponds to *sukshma-sharira*. This is the beginning of a process that renders one's body subtle; what ensues is a particular feeling of freshness and lightness. The tamasic element begins to be substituted by the tejasic element (*tejas* = radiating energy).

In a later phase of the same nocturnal and morning contemplation, the light should eventually be turned into warmth. This warmth, as one approaches *samyama*, should dissipate and leave as the only residue, in a cold brilliance, a bare, solar, absolute "I am."[20]

In the practice with prana it is important to try to gradually feel this warmth within the whole body, during inspiration and retention (more or less prolonged) of breath. The texts say that one should feel prana, the inner breath, as a tingling sensation on the palms of the hands and on the soles of the feet.[21] In the context of pranic sensation of one's body, the special objects of practice are the five *vayus*, currents or breaths, which I discussed in Chapter IV. Obviously, for this kind of experience it is necessary to be in contact with a depository of the corresponding traditional teachings. The definitions of the five *vayus* in the texts are complicated and often divergent, and therefore it is difficult to adopt a corresponding sadhana. The teachings concerning the sushumna, ida, and pingala, which I shall introduce later, are more univocal.

In some Tibetan yoga texts dealing with the experience of the "bright light" (*hodgsal*), one may find an intensification of practice through the contemplation of the nocturnal sun. This experience corresponds to the experience of the subtle state, which is encountered "in the interval between the end of the experience of the waking state and the beginning of the sleeping state." When ready to go to sleep, one must assume the "lion posture," which was also recommended by early Buddhism. In it, one lies on the right side. With the mind, one must move to the middle seat, corresponding to the heart.[22] In this seat one should be open to every reflection from the outside world, every image, every residual thought, until one reaches a state of calm concentration. The procedure outlined in the Tantric Tibetan texts is very complex and consists of several visualizations. First is the visualization of Shakti, which one should identify with one own's body. Next is the visualization of a four-petaled lotus flower in the heart, with the five mantras inscribed, the first in the middle, the others on the four petals (in order to position these sacred syllables correctly, the apprentice, facing north, will put AH on the northern petal, NU on the eastward petal, TA on the southward petal, and RA on the westward petal). The letters must be well written, bright, and shining. When sleep approaches, the calm and concentrated mind will go from one mantra to the next, and finally it will settle in the middle, on HUM, journeying along the Tibetan sign, moving from the bottom upward, and eventually landing in the little crescent and in the circle located at its upper corner; this circle, in this graphic symbol, represents *shunya*, "emptiness" or transcendence.[23] All of the mantras are visualized in the form of Tibetan letters and not in their transcription in the Western alphabet. Whether they have any objective effectiveness or not is strictly contingent on the level of spiritual awareness found in a Tibetan person.

The unanimous consent is that the bright light is found in the middle seat. The text to which I just referred calls the ensuing change of state, when sleep supervenes, "ignition," and calls the point of deep sleep, which corresponds to a further change of state, "completion." If consciousness could follow all these phases, it too would experience that absolute light which dazzles after death.[24] The state of ignition mentioned in the text visibly corresponds to the warm phase, which we indicated as that into which runs, through intensification, the bright perception of the subtle state.

A more simplified practice, which a Tantric Buddhist text indicates, consists in imagining one own's body as the body of Buddha Vajrasattva (whose substance is *vajra*, the "diamond thunderbolt") and in focusing the mind on the calm, empty state when one is about to fall asleep. It is interesting to notice the counterpart at the time of the awakening: in it, one should evoke "Shiva's two-sided drum," which echoes in the middle of the sky, proclaiming the words of power of the twenty-four heroes (divine figures of the Tibetan pantheon). When one emerges from the sleep state "in this state of the divine body," each surrounding thing should be considered as a sign or symbol (mandala) of itself, as Vajrasattva. A cosmic and powerful feeling arises as a consequence of practice when it is successful in establishing a communication of the waking consciousness with the superindividual consciousness that is buried in the sleeping state. This is not without relation to the formulation found in another text, which talks about the "shining of a bright light over the path followed during the day." This shining represents the insertion of the luminous, subtle consciousness in the various forms of sadhana. At that point the flux of mental formations stops and generates enlightened moments. One text describes the "unobscured, primordial condition of the mind, which shineth in interval between the cessation of one thought-formation and the birth of the next."[25]

Having previously considered teachings and practices concerning the body, I will now explain the meaning of the so-called asanas that are found in yoga. These are postures conferring to the body maximum stability and producing a feeling of well-being, so that one may retain them for a long time, remaining still, without effort and without getting tired. There are many asanas—the texts mention thirty of them. The most employed ones are *padma-asana* and *siddha-asana*. The latter differs from the former in that in *padma-asana* the feet, instead of simply lying one upon the other, are intertwined; the right foot rests on the left thigh, next to the groin, with the sole facing upward; the left foot rests on the right thigh, in an analogous way. Usually asanas are associated with mudras, signs or gestures that are given the meaning of "seals" (this is the literal meaning of the term *mudra*). Two mudras often associated with the two aforesaid asanas are (1) the gesture of the hands resting on the knees with the tip of the thumb touching the tip of the index finger, thus forming a circle, while the other fingers are extended; and (2) the hands are overlapping, horizontally, the right hand over the left, at the height of the navel, palms facing upward. Sometimes the term *mudra* is used as if synonymous with *asana*. There are three kinds of asanas; a coarse *(sthula)* mudra, a subtle *(sukshma)* mudra, and a supreme *(para)* mudra. The first is executed with the aid of physical limbs; in the second, a "word of power" (mantra) matches the gesture; the last is a seal that is realized even in its metaphysical substance. In the Bhavonopanishad (21–24) various mudras (= asanas) are associated with various chakras, or occult centers, more on which later.[26]

When I said that asanas are natural, pleasant, and effortless body postures, this must be understood in a relative sense. They may become so once the subject gets used to them, which may take a long time (especially for people who are not Indians, since people from India are accustomed to using similar postures even in ordinary life). The most important aspect in the employment of asanas and especially of mudras is a ritualistic and magical one.

First of all, asana may be considered a further development of a preliminary discipline, which consists in the suppression of unnecessary and random movements and in the full control of one's nerves and muscles. The yogin eliminates fluttering and disorderly thoughts (which are the first two stages of *chitta*), as well as any instinctive, untidy gesture, stemming from a natural desire to communicate.[27] He is reserved and carries no trace on his face of either thoughts or feelings, by virtue of exercising a total control of the facial muscles until he reaches the typically Aryan imperturbability of a statue.

Asanas are designed to promote a similar imperturbability in the entire body. This is not all. When it is said that asanas may be grasped in their true nature only through a guru, a spiritual teacher, it is implied that what really matters in them is the meaning of the gesture and the symbolic-ritualistic meaning of the posture. This is because through it, as Mircea Eliade correctly remarked, man tends to incarnate a god, to become transformed into its image, if not almost into its statue, or to reproduce a given aspect of it. Thus asanas are not without relation to the Tantric yoga habit of identifying one's body with the body of a given deity *(devata)* at the beginning of every practice session. The starting point is a vivified and somewhat magical image, which the bodily gesture ritually reproduces. On this basis, in the body's stillness there is something almost magical,[28] while various relationships between the pranic currents in the body and the forces found in nature are reproduced in the various postures. The "seal," in this context, represents the closing of a circuit, which determines a specific fluid state. Also, this theory of the asanas has a parallel in the hieratic stillness attested to in several ancient Western traditions. In the doctrine concerning the ancient Egyptian kingship, for instance, stability and stillness (expressed by the hieroglyphic *ded*) were conceived as a real, supernatural fluid flowing within the king's veins. In the classical mysteries *thronismos*, the ritual of sitting perfectly still on a throne was so important as to present close ties with initiation and with identification with the god.[29] In yoga, too, these ideas can be found, both as a gesture of the body, expressing an inner meaning, and as a higher meaning that animates and magically supports a gesture of the body.

This applies also to some aspects of mudras, in which case the term *gesture* has a more specific meaning, since the term *mudra* may also designate an action, a particular operation, that is considered in its unity and always in terms of a "seal."

· VII ·

THE VIRGIN:
RELEASE FROM BONDAGE

In Tantrism the practice of yoga in the strict sense of the word is competence of the divya type. Dhyana-yoga treatises are used to combine disciplines fostering meditation and concentration with some rules of life. The latter should not be understood according to the Western sense of moral laws. Their actual purpose is to avert any factors that may trouble or upset the soul and distract it from practice. The articulations of classical yoga, despite their mental or intellectual character, are not abstract and impractical disciplines. Unification of the mind requires unification of the soul; it cannot be achieved unless the soul is calm and trouble free. Such is the practical goal of a life-style that by a superficial observer may be considered to conform to moral rules. Classical yoga celebrates the brahmacharya state, consisting in sexual abstinence, among other things, since sex was considered one of the soul's main upsetting factors.

Very different is the orientation of the intermediate level of the viras' and kaulas' orders, since they are endowed with a rajas nature, inclined to action. The vira is given to the practice of *icchashuddhi*, a discipline promoting purification of the will. A pure will is a naked, transcendent will, capable of self-determination, which is beyond all antithetical values and all pairs of opposites. The ethics followed by viras and kaulas consists in the breaking and the overcoming of the bonds (pasha) characterizing the inferior, worldly person (pashu). A double symbolism has been associated to the corresponding task.

The first symbol is that of the mythological god Heruka, "who is without clothes" (this is also one of Shiva's characteristics).[1] The second symbol is that of the virgin (*kumari*), of Shakti as Uma, "no one's bride." It is said, "The power of the will is Uma, the Virgin." The vira must have the virgin; he has to forcibly strip her of all her clothes and rape her on her throne,[2] which means he has to take possession of and to incorporate the elementary nature of power. But in order to be able to do this he must walk on a long, rugged path.[3] The following are details on how that is accomplished. The Tantras contain several lists of pasha from which the vira must free himself in the course of his journey. I will outline the main pasha listed in the Kularvana-Tantra (X, 90) and add some clarifications.

SYMPATHY (*DAYA*)

Daya is the inclination to allow oneself to be moved and troubled by other people's sufferings and misfortunes. As "compassion for all living things" (in the West this virtue goes under the name "humanitarianism"), which in other Hindu spiritualities was considered a positive and meritorious attitude, *daya* is considered in Tantrism to be a bond (pasha). By so doing, the Tantras do not mean to idealize spiritual callousness and insensitive selfishness. To begin with, no mercy should be shown toward one's own self (enough for the charge of selfishness). Also, we are dealing here with a discipline that is obviously not meant for people given to mawkish sentimentality. In some cases emancipation requires a certain degree of harshness or relentlessness. After all, *daya* should not be equated with *karuna*, which is proper to a different plane and to the body of preliminary disciplines examined in this context. In fact, the ultimate, positive overcoming of the bond of individuality necessarily involves an openness that allows one to be in tune with other beings, but in a way that is free from sentimental perturbations, that is, at a superpersonal, objective level.

DELUSION (*MOHA*)

The pasha of delusion derives from a life-style that is inconsistent, without a center, and constantly gravitating around external factors to which the empirical subject draws its sense of identity: hence hope and its counterpart, delusion, which take place when one's hopes and goals are not fulfilled, and when one's expectations are not met. The vira rescinds this bond and purifies his will, since external circumstances do not dishearten him but always find him active and invulnerable. Obviously, this rescindment requires a flexible and agile will, if one is to let go and to subsequently keep going, without dwelling on negative factors and thus allowing them to break one's spirit. In a wider context than a mere strengthening of the will, besides the capability of accepting all things as unavoidable, it is a matter of understanding. It is taught that delusions, adversities, personal tragedies and failures, even catastrophes may play the role of a hidden guru, of a spiritual teacher *sui generis;* they may be interpreted as signs to discern the right path.

SHAME AND SIN (*LAJJA*)

The vira does not take other people's criticisms into consideration. The positive and negative comments about him made by the society in which he lives do not affect him. He is beyond shame and honor. He does not accept judgment according to the standards of ordinary society, but he does not hesitate to subject himself to the criticisms of an authoritative guru of the order to which he belongs. It is improper to speak of "sin" in this context. The notion of sin, as it has been understood by the Judeo-Christian tradition, is not found in Asia nor in the Aryan world, in either its Eastern or Western hemispheres. The latter knows the concept of "fault" rather than "sin," in the sense of contamination, or impurity (an impurity that is almost physical, as in ancient Greece). When sin is reduced to the notion of guilt, it does not have a moral connotation, but it rather denotes a wrong action, performed in an irrational frame of mind. Earlier we learned that according to the Hindu doctrine of karma, he who violates his own dharma does not become a "sinner" but rather endures the consequences of his own actions. In this context, the pasha to be overcome could be identified with a "guilty conscience." The vira's will is purified, since he does not allow thoughts of guilt to torment him. He takes responsibility for his wrongdoing without apologizing. He leaves his faults behind, animated by a renewed and stronger determination to err no more.

FEAR (*BHAYA*)

Tantrism attributes particular value to this bond and to its overcoming. More than any other it characterizes ordinary humans

95

(pashus); likewise its absence characterizes true viras. This is not an ordinary physical and animal-like fear, but rather a kind of fear that arises from deep levels within one's being, and which may manifest itself in supernatural experiences. In Appendix One of this book we shall learn how, in the after-death experiences described in the Bardo Thödol, fear may preclude the achievement of liberation by preventing a person from identifying with terrifying and over-whelming forces. Thus in some ancient Western and Indian rites, special ordeals were prepared for the apprentice. In order to complete them successfully one needed to conquer fear and disgust and to demonstrate spiritual courage. During these trials ceremonial and magical means were employed. We may presume that Tantrism, with a similar intent, sometimes employed magical practices that originally had a black-magic ring to them. Such, for instance, is the practice of *shavasana* ("dead posture"). He who practices sadhana is supposed to go at night to a deserted house, a mountaintop, or a cemetery. There he must sit astride a corpse that has been laid on its belly, facing north. He must draw on the corpse's back a graphic symbol (yantra), usually an inverted triangle, representing Shakti. At this point he evokes elementary forces by reciting mantras and by projecting prana in the corpse with the purpose of animating it (*pranapratishtha*) and of producing a temporary incarnation of the evoked force. If the rite is successful, this force actually manifests itself in the corpse, whose head will then spin around and speak to the apprentice. The apprentice must be able to impose his will right away on the "ghost." This practice is considered terrifying and most dangerous. It is by far the gloomiest practice mentioned in the Tantras, and it is influenced by the demonic substratum of aboriginal populations.[4]

DISGUST (*GHRINA*)

According to a Tantric text, "All the means employed must be experienced without disgust, concupiscence, or attachment."[5]

FAMILY, KINSHIP, CLAN (*KULA*)

Kinship ties are bonds of a natural and affective type, most cherished by what in Western countries may be called a bourgeois life-style. Because of what has been said so far, it is difficult to picture a vira as a parent, a spouse, or an obedient child. In his own way he is a bona fide ascetic, no less than a sannyasin, who, according to the traditional Hindu doctrine of the four ashramas, is a person who has become free from family and caste-related duties. The Tantric apprentice's detachment is rather an inner event.

CASTE (VARNA)

According to Indo-Aryan tradition, a caste corresponds to an individual differentiated nature, and to the body of laws (dharma) one should follow. In the Left-Hand Path, however, dharma is seen as a limitation, or as a conditioning to be overcome. Purification of the will requires that no given existential situation, legacy, personal relationship, or inner law should become a bond. *Attivarna*, the suppression of various caste-system prerogatives (suppression from above and not from below, as it is advocated by "champions" of human rights or by liberal democrats), was likewise an ascetic's privilege. Despite the situation characteristic of the last age, Kali Yuga, which is one marked by dissolution, Tantrism does not accept any caste limitations. It shares the early Buddhist perspective according to which one who is picking firewood does not care from what tree it came. Likewise, it does not matter to what caste a person pursuing absolute liberation belongs. Obviously, this is a case of apparent "democracy." The capability of effectively walking on the path produces differentiations among people that are more clean-cut and real than the ones due to caste membership, especially when the latter have lost their original and legitimate foundation.

PRECEPTS, RITES, VARIOUS OBSERVANCES AND INTERDICTIONS (SILA)

Sila are the bonds of morality and of social conformity. Antinomianism and the release of the will from all laws are in Tantrism carried to their utmost consequences, to the point where "one should feel able to commit incest with one's mother and sister." When it comes to sayings like that, however, it should not be forgotten that we are dealing with a formulation of the highly symbolic, multifaceted language that we shall encounter in later chapters. As in the case of "philosophical incest," which is advocated by the Western Hermetic-alchemical tradition, we may refer to an esoteric interpretation that plays down such alarming precepts. The "mother" one should feel free to possess is Parashakti, the primordial force from which everything originates; she is portrayed as the Mother or as the Virgin. When instead of Parashakti we consider the female Shakti, Shiva's counterpart, we must conclude that the two are "brother and sister," since they are generated from the same source point (Parashakti). Thus their sexual union— a fundamental principle of Tantrism—is actually an act of incest. Such a symbolic interpretation, however, is still too theoretical in the context of the purification of the will. It was shunned, for instance, by the Aghori sect, which in the course of the sexual rituals celebrated in Durga's honor purposely practiced incest. Symbolic interpretations were also rejected by those Tantric *chakras* (initiatory chains) who believed that it should not matter if the woman to be employed in *maithuna* happened to be a sister or a daughter.

The essence of *pashaniroda*, the release from bondage, is the achievement of an inner state in which the vira feels that there is nothing he is not able to do,[6] since *icchashuddhi*, the complete purification of the will, the possession of the Virgin, has led him beyond every antithesis, into neutral ground. He will feel "equally in regard to himself, friends and foes; pleasure and pain; heaven and hell; good and evil; contempt and praise; day and night; poverty and wealth; a prostitute and his own mother; wife and daughter; reality and dreams; what is perennial and what is ephemeral."[7]

Once the pasha have been cut, the vira becomes *avredhuta*, one who is washed from all dirt. He is "naked," like the divine archetype represented by the Egyptian god Heruka.

Quite frankly, the suspicion may arise that these are nothing but phony cover-ups and empty words, and that what is falsely believed to be liberation or purification in reality is the removal of obstacles preventing one from unleashing his animal instincts with no restraints whatsoever. We cannot rule this out, but again I must remind the readers of the saying "A sharpened edge of a razor, a difficult path is this!" At this point some considerations are in order. First of all we must presuppose a thorough examination of one's motives and inclinations, whether this work is carried out by the individual or by a guru. For instance, if one finds himself to be hard-hearted, the discipline that will successfully help him to achieve a neutral state and a naked will is not the destruction of the *daya* (sympathy) bond—since its destruction will strengthen that disposition—but rather the contrary. Likewise, if one admits to a hidden attraction toward a young and beautiful sister, incest will not help him to wrest the will from *sila's* bonds and to overcome them.

Second, the removal of pashas should not be considered apart from a larger context including other disciplines. Here, cheating oneself is next to impossible. One of the disciplines is obedience. It is not a coincidence that the viras' doctrine, which views the adept as *svecchakari* ("he who does as he pleases"), teaches that the disciple must surrender himself as an inanimate object to his spiritual teacher and obey his orders without questioning whether they are reasonable, fair, or humane.[8] There are many stories about endless, inexorable, and exasperating trials to which various disciples submitted themselves, following the instructions of their teachers. Today the house that Milarepa had to build, destroy, and rebuild for endless years is still standing. The meaning of all this is the following. To comply perfectly with someone else's will, without recriminating or beating about the bush, is a good way to shape the will of an insufficiently strong individual, and to make it capable of absolute self-determination outside the binding tendencies and inclinations due to karmic or regular conduct. The ultimate purpose is not to give up one's will, but to purify it, to increase its powers, and to individualize it, thus making it absolute and truly autonomous.

A parallel may be drawn with the ancient Islamic order of the Ishmaelites. This order comprised an initiatic hierarchy of seven levels. In the higher levels the guiding principle was analogous to the Tantric viras' and kaulas' principle, "nothing exists, everything is permitted." In order to be admitted to the higher levels, candidates were first required to go through the lower levels, in which unconditional obedience was the norm. This obedience was so radical that in some cases it required giving up one's life without any valid reason if the supreme leader of the order so commanded. A similar episode occurred when its leader, Sheik al-Gabir, met with the count of Champagne during the Crusades.

It is clear by now that the release from bondage is not a matter of removing, with the excuse of pursuing initiatory practices, those obstacles preventing one from unleashing one's samsaric nature. This does not affect what I have expounded about the purification of passions through passions themselves. That is a different issue altogether.

That impulses arising from the deepest recesses of one's being are kept under control is attested to by the special attention turned to the so-called karmic body. This body corresponds to all the elements, under the form of samskaras, assumed by an individual from prenatal samsaric currents. The presupposition for this body's absolute purification consists in separating the will from such a body and in making the will autonomous from it.

I would like at this point to refer to something other than yogic procedures. There is a practice that is employed by Buddhist Tantrism in pursuit of the same goal. It is difficult to take this practice out of its socio-geographical context.

This practice is called *chöd*, a Tibetan word that means "to cut off," and more specifically, to cut the bond represented by the karmic body. It takes place in the context of ceremonial magic, with the participation of dark, demonic factors. The inner strength required to go through it is also designated as the "indomitable courage." Committed to the goal of getting rid of all hopes and fears, the person undergoing the ritual evokes, with the aid of magic, various elemental forces, ordering them to devour his no-longer-needed samsaric body, so that the samsaric I may be released, the debt paid, and the conditioning overcome. What is left is the I's nucleus and sheer power. Following the magical phase of the sacrifice, to which the ritual imparts a dramatic and terrifying overtone, what follows is the knowledge of the void, bringing to an end the consumption of the samsaric-karmic legacy. In the course of it, one realizes that the idea of sacrifice is a bond caused by ignorance, since there is nothing to be abandoned and nobody to give things back to, because nothing really exists as other.[9] It is said that the ritualistic-sacrificial evocation of *chöd* may sometimes be substituted by purely inner operations of high contemplation. On the one hand, the norm is that one who has begun such rituals must go through them without help. On the other hand, constant mention is made of the triple danger intrinsic in these magical-ritualistic practices: illness, derangement, and even death.

When *icchashuddhi*, the purification of the will, is pursued in any of the ways so far described, which are typical of initiatory Left-Hand Tantric practices, a critical level is reached. At this level[10] one is practically deprived of all ordinary, everyday motivations, thus becoming "paralyzed" and without support. This level, however, is a crucial one. It can be overcome only by employing a self-determined strength and by being endowed with the pure, unblemished principle of the Virgin, represented by control over *maya-shakti*, which is the centrifugal energy of desire and of samsara. A reference is made to the passage of the Bhagavad-Gita in which Krishna proposes himself as an example to Arjuna; even though the process of creation is completed in him, he still acts by dominating his own nature. Thus the vira may consider himself *sui securus* ("certain about himself"); he may be certain of his invulnerability when pursuing any experience recommended by the Tantric Way.

· VIII ·

THE EVOCATIONS:
THE NAMES OF POWER

While popular forms of Tantrism indulged in the devotional cult (*shakti-puja*) and in the worship (*shakti-upasana*) of the goddess Shakti, higher forms of Tantrism practiced instead the contemplation of Shakti (*shakti-dhyana*). *Shakti-dhyana* consists of two phases, which are influenced by two sayings derived from the Upanishadic tradition by replacing *brahman* with *Shakti*: "Everything is Shakti," and "I am this Shakti."

The first phase of the contemplation of Shakti deals with the interiorization and the realization of the Shaktic worldview, which I have already expounded. This phase is characterized not by mere speculation but by the attempt to lead the apprentice to an experience of the objective dimension of reality. This experience can be defined as a magical-symbolic perception of the world, which allows the individual to live and to act in a nature, a light, a space and time, and a series of causes and effects that are qualitatively different from those that characterize the natural environment inhabited by contemporary humanity. In the course of history a modification has taken place concerning not only the forms of subjective thought but also the fundamental categories of objective

101

experience. We may say that maya's veil has become increasingly thicker and that the hiatus between I and not-I has widened considerably. The two main consequences of this process are the perception of the universe in terms of pure outwardness and the removal of the existential foundation of the previous living and sacred worldview. Modern science has built its theories on this lifeless and superficial exteriority.

Shakti-dhyana's goal is to retrieve the primordial living perception of the world. The first phase of dhyana is based on the principle of correspondence; every phenomenon, thing, or state is associated with an immaterial power, with a being, or with a deity (*devata*).[1] The second phase is based on the principle of identity: "Not only do these phenomena, things, or states of being correspond to these powers; they *are* these very powers." In the course of sadhana the combined action of sadhana's various aspects is supposed to lead the apprentice from the first phase, which consists of the foreboding of supersensible presences, to some sort of psychic perception (*ritambhara*). This perception is gradually stripped of external elements and processes until it reaches a final stage, in which formless "roots" (hence the term "emptiness," *shunya* or *shunyata*), corresponding to essences,[2] are eventually perceived.

Evocative procedures of a ceremonial and theurgic type, which were well known in the ancient Western world as well, may facilitate the disclosure of the silent outwardness of reality by breaking through it and acting in a violent and dramatic way, even though the effects may be short-lived. Dhyana, which may develop into a true *samyama*, is based on an aspect of nature that is often associated with a graphic symbol (yantra, mandala), or with a formula (mantra), or with a mudra, or with a deity (*devata*). Yantras and mandalas, as I have said, are not abstract and general symbols, but rather the *signaturae rerum*. They are related to the forms that are assumed by various powers on a subtle or causal plane; in other words, they facilitate the perception of the living meanings and of the forces underlying the phenomena, processes, or appearances found in nature. I have also indicated that the term *seal* (mudra). may be referred to the ritual postures assumed by various divinities. These postures have a "form [gestalt] of the gesture," which, once it has been understood, is believed to have an enlightening and revelatory power.

We thus arrive at the varieties of *shakti-dhyana*, whose object is the image of a deity (*devata*, shakti, *dakini*, etc.), which may be the same found in traditional cults. Here the magical power of the imagination plays an even greater role than in other practices. In Tantrism there are complex procedures that include, in the case of some Tibetan schools, the so-called creation of the gods. Hindu Tantrism, when its object is a material image (a painting or a statue), pursues the pranic animation of this image. The *devata,* or shakti, or *dakini,* is "evoked" by means of the "body," which consists in a vivified mental image projected into it. The act that sanctions the "real presence" (*avahana*) comes after the dismissal of the evoked force (*visarjana*).[3] The reference to prana implies that the evocation requires mental and psychic intermediaries, since a force in the subtle plane cannot directly manifest itself into something material. The practice of magical-fluid animation of various images can also be found in other traditions, especially in the Egyptian tradition.[4]

In yoga the vivification and transformation of prana sometimes take place through subtle energies that emanate from the yogin. This happens during the state of his absolute, prolonged bodily stillness, as he focuses with his mind on this image. In some circumstances, however, some techniques inducing excitement are employed, such as an orgasm, obtained in an adequately supervised sexual union. In other cases, the image is charged through a collective ritual performed in a Tantric circle.

In Tibetan Buddhism the essential instrument employed during practice is *vajra-chitta,* the unchangeable mind, which gradually feeds the fire of the imagination. A distinction should be made between *jnani-devata* and *bhakta-devata.* The former corresponds to a mental image; the latter to an image produced by an ecstatic rapture and known on a religious plane as "adoration." This is the basis on which the god is "created." Also, the texts say that the *devatas* created by the mind are as real as living *devatas.* That claim must be understood in the following sense: by virtue of the principle of analogy, the visualization and animation processes are confused with the process of a real, objective evocation. Thus, because of the similarity between the two, the created image attracts a power that transforms it into the body of its own temporary manifestation.

This is the first, "creative" or "speculative," phase of the process. The second phase corresponds to the practical goals pursued during practice. All things considered, the real goal is the experience of power, by virtue of which one is able to overcome the world of external phenomena. The act of evoking and then dismissing a *devata* or a shakti corresponds to the emerging and to the subsequent dimming of such an enlightening experience. Thus, during the second phase of the contemplative process, one aims at eliminating any duality and at identifying with the deity that has been evoked. Usually the method employed consists in going from the image of the *bhakti-devata* to its mantra; from the mantra to *bija*; from *bija* to "emptiness" (*shunya*, the dimension of transcendence) and then to *vajra*, where the *devata* produces a purely spiritual experience. In kundalini yoga and in Vajrayana's yoga these "identifications" take place within the body's secret centers (chakras); in the chakras, the *devatas*, the shaktis, and *dhyani-buddhas* (buddhas who personify in their gestures—mudras—the various phases of the realization process) are known according to their true nature. At a given moment, the various parts of sadhana condition and integrate one another.

This does not prevent the principle of identification from characterizing a phase of *shakti-dhyana* during a peculiar Tantric ritual. The bottom line of this ritual consists in the evocation of a *devata* or of a shakti, and in actualizing their real presence in the form of a material image. This material image is eventually identified with one's body. The procedure is the same: a divine image is evoked, fixed, and roused in a specific mudra (a magical-symbolic gesture that expresses its essence) and in its traditional and esoteric attributes. After that, the apprentice imagines his own body and his person to be the deity's. In Tibetan Tantrism this is but a preliminary ritual, which is also used in yoga as a prelude to spiritual actions. A text provides some further details.

The basic image is that of the *vajra-yogini*, the naked Virgin. She is a goddess made of *vajra*, whose body is bright red and whose attributes are more or less the same as Kali's. The apprentice identifies with her and imagines her body to be the size of his own body. In the course of the visualization process, he expands this shining figure with his mind and imagines her to be as big as a house, then as big as a hill, then as vast as the universe. Then, in reverse, he imagines her smaller and smaller, until she is reduced to the size of a seed, still having all the limbs and parts sharply defined. In both cases he is supposed to visualize every single detail. This rhythm of expansion and contraction is somehow related to the practice of reabsorption of the cosmic prana, more on which later. If such a practice is the prelude to yogic actions, the goddess's shape should be visualized as being shining and internally vacuous, almost as if it consisted of a mere transparent and luminous membrane. Likewise, the inside of one's body is perceived as empty; within this formless space the magical visualizations are supposed to take place. These visualizations, in turn, act on different pranic currents and generate various degrees of enlightenment.[5] Such practices, if followed thoroughly, are not exempt from dangers, since they could induce various forms of frenzy.

As I have said, beyond the various powers, divinities, and shaktis underlying phenomena and things, one should gradually come to realize the fundamental unity of all these energies, according to the first of the two Upanishadic sayings: "Truly, all of this is Shakti." Contemplation, thereafter, gives way to the phase of identification: "Between this Shakti and me there is no difference whatsoever," "I am nothing but Shakti herself." Such is the leitmotif of the Tantric cult at the contemplative level. Naturally, this may merely represent a preliminary state of mind. One text says:

I am Her [Shakti]: this idea will eventually lead one to be transformed into Her. . . . Let the apprentice do everything, from early in the morning to late at night, with the awareness of the *devata's* immanent presence. Such a habit will develop a divine frame of mind through which the apprentice will achieve various siddhis. Only he who has acquired such a frame of mind will become a *siddha.* . . . The theme of contemplation is that nothing in the world exists outside of Her; the mass of her spirit, her fire, and her radiating energy *(tejas)* fills the universe. The apprentice who acquires this awareness will move freely like a god while remaining on earth. Despite having a human body, in truth he is not a man, but a god. . . . There is nothing that he ought to worship. He deserves people's worship, but nobody deserves his.[6]

Another Tantric practice is the so-called *nyasa,* which is a preliminary stage of what in Vajrayana constitutes the arousal of the *vajra-rupa.* The term *nyasa* comes from the verb "to put." It is a process of invocation of real presences, whose object no longer is the body as a whole, but individual parts, spots, and organs, according to the Tantric principle: "The body is the temple of the deity, and the living being is Sadashiva himself." Through *nyasa* one induces or awakens various deities and shaktis in various parts of the body, especially in the so-called vital points. The texts distinguish several *nyasas. Kara-nyasa* consists in touching the fingers in order to make the hand "come to life"; *anga-nyasa* focuses on the main members of the body, commencing from the heart and ending with the hands.[7] From another point of view, there are internal creative or "dissolving" *nyasas*, each endowed with more articulations. Beyond such a distinction, this process too has a ritual and a *samyama* aspect, the latter being a contemplative realization based on mantra. Sometimes they are expressed in sayings like this: "AM [the mantra] and the life [prana] of the god X are present here."[8] In this, as well as in other cases, the degree of the ritual action's effectiveness is directly proportional not only to the spiritual and initiatic levels reached by the apprentice but also to his dignity and to his consecrating virtue, of which he must be aware and in which he must have an unwavering faith. During *nyasa* this action consists in putting the hand on or in pointing the finger at different parts of the body, while pronouncing a mantra and simultaneously realizing, through the mind, the real presence of various *devatas*. If the hand has been "made alive" by a shakti, the part that has been touched will come to life: divine life will flow into it. Then the material organ, made of *vajra* and the sattva guna, would begin to awaken. Following individual isolated impositions in the course of the ritual, the hand is moved over the entire body as if to rub over its surface the divine fluid; finally, a transformation of the human figure is imagined or visualized. A dark man ridden with guilt is burned in the spiritual fire, and his place is taken by a new body made of light, which is exalted and rendered subtle by the "nectar of joy," which springs forth from the divine couple's intercourse. This new body is also thought to be made of mantra, which is to say, of *vajra*. These teachings have a counterpart in magical Western traditions. I again quote Agrippa, who, in a chapter of his *De occulta philosophia* aptly entitled "Of the members of God, and of their influence on our human members," wrote: "If a man capable of the divine influence do make any member of his body clean and free from filthiness, then it becomes the *habitale* and proper seat of the secret limb of God, and of the virtue to which the same name is ascribed."[9]

Agrippa goes on to say: "These are the great and hidden mysteries concerning which it is not lawful to publish more." A more direct reference, which characterizes the ultimate goal of the procedure, is found in the hieratic-initiatory tradition of ancient Egypt; various practices attempted to make all the body's organs "talk"; this, obviously, is the equivalent to the arousal of ecstatic and magical states.

Usually *nyasa* is associated to another practice (*bhutashuddhi*), or the purification of the elements and of matter, which constitutes *nyasa*'s premise. This practice has a purely inner character, and it somehow prefigures what will take place in the course of yoga in its *laya* aspect. Its basis consists in imagining the series of subtle centers located along the axis of the spinal cord. The lowest of these centers corresponds to the earth, while the others refer to the remaining elements and to the higher tattvas, all the way to *parasamvid*, which is located on the top of the head. I will discuss these centers at greater length in Chapter X. *Bhutashuddi* consists in the mental realization of each element's dissolution and transformation into a hierarchically higher element, which in turn is considered subtler and purer. This is achieved by shifting the mental fire of the visualization process from one center to the next.[10] If the inner sensitivity is sharpened, the effect will be similar to a circuit's breakdown into a series of states, or degrees of power, until it reaches a certain level of saturation and vibratility. This level facilitates the following operation, consisting in imposition through the *nyasa*. I said that *bhutashuddi* is a prefiguration because, allegedly, the process of the ascending reabsorption of the elements is real only at the level of kundalini yoga. The same goes for the bodily organs' "divinization" through *nyasa*.

The following details about *bhutashuddi* are found in the Mahanirvana-Tantra. The earth is dissolved into water; water into fire; fire into air; air into ether. This takes place as each of the senses of the body is dissolved into another, in the following order: touch, smell, taste, sight, and hearing; hearing is dissolved into *ahamkara-tattva*; the latter into buddhi; buddhi into prakriti (that is, into shakti); prakriti into *brahman*. One must then proceed to imagine a dark man, situated in the left side of the abdominal cavity, as a sinful body. The following stages of this practice include pranayama, the correct way of breathing. One must inhale sixteen times from the left nostril, while evoking YAM, the air's mantra. One must visualize it as engulfed in smoke and think that, in this fashion, the dark man's substance will dry up. While retaining breath for sixty-four repetitions of RAM (the fire's mantra, which is situated in the chakra at the level of the navel), one must imagine that this act is bringing about the destruction of the dark man's substance. Finally, during an exhalation lasting thirty-two times, one must evoke the white *varna-bija*, the "heavenly waters" mantra, which is situated in the forehead. One must imagine the pouring out of a fluid from the burned-up dark body, which generates a new divine body. Such a body will be consolidated by visualizing LAM, the earth's yellow mantra, which is located in the *muladhara-chakra*, and by staring at it calmly and firmly. What follows is *nyasa*. It "infuses into this new body the life of the Devi" and it makes a macrocosm out of the apprentice's body.[11] The formula SA'HAM ("I am her") seals the double ritual.

I have frequently mentioned the word *mantra*. At this time it is appropriate to provide some further details. *Mantra* may designate a simple liturgical formula, an invocation, or a prayer. If by the term we designate a formula or a magical syllable, then the employment of mantras dates back to the Vedic period (specific references to mantras are found in the Atharva-Veda). It plays such a major role in Tantrism that some have called it the Mantrayana, the "Path of the Mantra." The most interesting aspect is the metaphysical development (especially in the Northern school) of the doctrine of the mantras, which can be connected with the doctrine of the tattvas. A wide development and a peculiar articulation was also given to the theory or theology of what in some ancient philosophies, and even in Alexandrian Christianity, was called *logos* (*verbum*, or the Word). In Tantric Buddhism the science of mantras corresponds to the second esoteric mystery (*guhya*), namely, to the transformation of the word into a *vajra* nature, or, to put it in other words, to the awakening of the "living word" made of power. Following the analogous awakening of the "living thought" and of the magical imagination (the first *guhya*), the third and final *guhya* consists in the arousal of the same *vajra* (diamond-thunderbolt) quality in the body.

The background theory may be summarized in the following way. Shakti and her manifestation are conceived as a sound or as a verb (*shabda, vak*); even the various phases of the cosmic development are also interpreted accordingly. The differentiation between Shiva and Shakti corresponds to the differentiation between the expression or expressive sound (*shabda*) and the meaning or object intended (*artha*). We may recall here the triple order of tattvas (pure, semipure, and impure) and its relationship with the "three worlds," with the three bodies (causal, subtle, and material), and with the three stages of atman. At the level of the first of the three orders, gemination has not yet reached a level whereby the "other" acquires an outward character. Therefore *artha* is not an object, but a pure meaning, or better, an object in the form of a meaning, as is the case of the process of forming human ideas. Something simple, endowed with a nature of pure light, puts the terms *shabda* and *artha* on the plane of *ishvara-tattva*, in the state where prajna and atman are conceived as pure affirmation (*anujna*). At the level of the semipure tattvas the differentiation and articulation processes begin to unfold. Also, the whole comprising the "letters," "syllables," or "sounds," which are included in the ineffable unity of the metaphysical "great dot" (*parabindu*), unfolds in distinct forms (the texts say that the "dot" eventually bursts open). These are the "subtle letters" or "causal letters," which correspond to the *devatas* and to the shaktis, namely, to the various powers of a *natura naturans;* they are called "little mothers" (*matrikas*), "seeds," and "roots" (*bijas*). A relationship could be established between the subtle letters and what Greek metaphysics called *logoi spermatikoi*, the Kabbala called "letters of light," and medieval magical speculation called *claviculae*. These do not exist in a material dimension; the "sounds" that are here being discussed cannot be heard; they are occult sounds (*avyaktarva-nada*), ways and "agglomerates" of immaterial power, *artha's* correlations being "lightning," or forms of light. The universe and every being are made of these sounds and letters. In Hindu doctrine, ether (*akasha*) is considered the substratum of every phenomenon. On the one hand, ether (which has nothing in common with the ether described by modern physics) is believed to be alive ("made of life," or of prana); on the other hand, its substance is believed to be "sound" or "word." The "seat" that corresponds to the doctrine of the three states is *tajasa*, which is blocked by sleep to ordinary man's consciousness.

Let us now deal with the plane of impure tattvas, which corresponds to the waking state and to the material world. The law of this world consists in an other being formed out of an I; this marks the passage from objectivity to subjectivity. Such a division is also found in the realm of words: on the one hand, there are *shabda* and *artha*, the name-voice, or the spoken language; on the other hand, there is the object signified (*rupa*) by the voice, which is external to it. We are now on the plane of contingent and particular beings. First of all, the relationship between word and object is no longer direct, but is now mediated, discursive, and conventional. The name no longer evokes an eternal meaning through an illumination, but evokes a mere material image, which is corruptible and perceived by the senses. The voice is now a material voice (*sthulashabda*). Secondly, through the power of *kankukas*, the contents of experience are nothing but the phenomena found in space and time. These phenomena are perceived by a finite consciousness, yet they depend on it for their manifestation. Even the name is now differentiated according to the multiplicity of languages. For instance, the word for fire in Sanskrit is *agni*, in Tibetan *me*, in Latin *ignis*, in German *feuer*. All these names evoke, not fire as such, but various representations of fire. Therefore, the so-called nominalist theory claims that the "universals" (general concepts) are nothing but mere verbal abstractions, lacking in content, since there is no such thing as "fire," but only this or that fire, which is perceived by the senses.

With this theory in the background, the mantras aim at restoring the word to a state in which the name no longer evokes the image of an object, but rather its power (shakti). In this state, the word no longer represents a noise produced by a certain individual, but rather represents the voice of the thing itself, as it reverberates outside the reach of human ears in the form of a cosmic language, or "language of the gods." After all, several traditions bear witness to the idea of a universal and essential language, in which everything has its natural, original, and eternal name, made of sacred and divine letters. According to Agrippa, these letters "are similar among all people, no matter what language they speak."[12] A reference to this phenomenon is found in the biblical myth of the tower of Babel and in the ensuing confusion of the languages. A mantra is, therefore, a word restored to its pristine state.

The faculties attributed to the mantras derive from the organic worldview of this doctrine, according to which the finite, material, and physical world is only a manifestation of the subtle, supersensuous, and transcendent world. It has been suggested that the tattvas do not dissolve into each other, but that they subsist simultaneously on their own planes—in the same way that the inner and outer aspects of an object coexist and are simultaneous. As in the human body all the gods and all the shaktis are present, likewise in the human language all the letters and names of the transcendent word are present in an occult way: hence a triple correspondence, which is at the basis of the doctrine of the mantras.

In the first place, there is a correspondence between the letters and syllables of a human alphabet, and the matrikas ("little mothers," "letters of light") and the bijas (the "syllables/seeds") of the subtle plane, in which the devatas and the shaktis are connected to corresponding bijas. Second, there is a certain connection of these letters and syllables to parts of the vital, subtle centers of the human organism, which are conceived as the seats of these powers, and as the creation of the powers manifested in the letters. Third, there is a correspondence of the letters with elemental powers of things, since the same principles, once the dualistic law of maya-shakti becomes operative, are manifested in both man and nature.

The Evocations: The Names of Power

As far as practice is concerned, the point of departure is represented by the so-called *sphota*, which is the object of various interpretations among different Hindu schools of thought. Generally speaking, *sphota* influences the evocative power of every word and every name. It is the phenomenon by virtue of which a given word (*shabda*) presents to the mind a specific image or suggests to it a specific meaning. In their interpretation of the *sphota*, the Tantras for the most part agree with the views expounded by Mimamsa, a Hindu darshana that distinguishes the material sound, produced by a vibration and by a clash of two objects—a "generated" and temporary sound—from an eternal and immaterial sound. The evocative power of a language and of a name derives from the fact that the audible material sound is only the form through which the other sound is manifested and expressed. The other sound, which essentially belongs to the plane of buddhi, is a determined and superindividual principle, to be found well beyond the duality of inner and outer and beyond the duality of concept (as idea or conversational notion) and reality. (This corresponds to the view according to which, for instance, in every combustion, a self-subsistent, uncreated, undifferentiated fire is manifested as a result of specific material causes.) *Sphota* is believed to be possible in reference to this plane, in which the voice still has the object in itself.

This implies that in every act of understanding there is, whether potentially or partially, an evocative power that is not confined exclusively to the sensory and dualistic order of things. Mantras are believed to be the support of such a reintegration. Having been handed down by an immemorial wisdom, the mantras are the *devatas'* names and the seminal and shaping forces in both nature and in the human body. They are hints of an "absolute language" or of a "divine language."

The Tantric texts are careful to specify that a mantra should not be confused with its expression through a material syllable or word, whether written or spoken, any more than a god should be mistaken for his image carved in wood or in stone. The mantra must be "awakened." The mental fire projected on it must consume the mantra's materiality and transform it into a subtle form "made of light." This is accomplished by inducing, on a higher plane, the phenomenon of *sphota*, or evocation—which suggests an opening or a blossoming (the literal meaning of the term *sphota* is "bursting forth"). Before all this, the mantra is "asleep"; it is a mere noise without any real powers. An explicit Tantric teaching says that if one does not know the meaning or the awakening of a mantra, it

THE YOGA OF POWER

remains inoperative, even if it is repeated a million times. The knowledge of the *devata* presiding over a mantra (*adhishthatri-devata*) is associated with the awakening of a mantra (*mantra-chaitanya*) and with the power that arouses it.[13]

The majority of the texts suggest that an indispensable requirement must be fulfilled before one ventures into this world; the mantras are not to be learned from books, but should rather be communicated orally and personally from a spiritual teacher in very specific circumstances. Only then will the disciple be able to sense the right direction to follow and to begin to pronounce with the "magical mind" (*vajra-chitta*) the mantra; in this case the mantra will be much more than just an unintelligible sound (the vast majority of mantras and *bijas*, unlike what some artificial and overly allegorical exegeses of the letters forming a mantra claim, do not have any meaning whatsoever, since they are mere sounds).

That having been said, the most frequently employed technique to awaken a mantra is its repetition (*japa*). This repetition at first is only verbal, and its object is the mantra in its dormant, coarse form. Later, the mantra is no longer repeated, even though its pronunciation lingers on. Eventually the repetition is purely mental (*manasa-japa*). At this level, the mantra is transformed from mere sound into an act of the spirit.

The technique of repetitions, which is found in several traditions, is twofold. In the first aspect, it acts as a sort of pratyahara; it helps to focus the mind, to dull the outer sensibility, and to awaken the inner sensibility through an active hypnosis. The second aspect is a magical one, and it refers to an intrinsic power that is attributed to the mantra. This action, to use a Catholic theological expression, is to a certain extent *ex opere operato*. The vibrations add up and are reverberated, thus affecting, through the subconscious, various forces and subtle centers of the body. The result is a progressive saturation that facilitates the mantra's awakening and opening. According to a Tantric image, *japa* is like shaking a person who is asleep until that person awakens and begins to move.

Analogously, the doctrine of the mantras may facilitate the intuitive comprehension of the relationship between the "three worlds" (the three seats, or the triple order of tattvas). Let us think of a book written in an unknown foreign language; skimming through the pages, we will see only a bunch of characters. We may compare this experience to the empirical experience of the material and phenomenal world, which common humanity perceives during the waking state. Conversely, if we could read or understand this foreign language, when hearing it, our mind would no longer stop at the characters, or at the sounds, but on the contrary would grasp its meaning directly and in depth. The first case applies to those who experience reality only in terms of physical exteriority; the second case applies to those who experience reality either in the function of the shaping forces that are at work in the subtle world or in the sounds and the corresponding "syllables/roots;" the third case applies to the experience of the causal world and of the pure tattvas. At this last level, the word is a living word and power. It is a word that commands physical reality, since in Hindu doctrine the physical vibrations are conceived as the tamasic and automatic appearance of subtle vibrations which in turn depend on various meanings. The command of those who have reached this supreme plane is like a thunderbolt that travels along the entire hierarchy, starting from the top until it reaches the vibrations at the very bottom, which shape matter. This is the so-called *vajra-vak*, the diamond-thunderbolt of the living word.

Thus Tantrism examines various dimensions of a word, in relation to the doctrines of kundalini and of the aforementioned centers in the human body (chakras). The spoken word is seen as the last echo or reflection of a deep process. In a text quoted by Arthur Avalon we read: "It is said that in the *muladhara* the 'air' (*Prana-vayu*) first appears. That 'air' acted upon by the effort of a person desiring to speak, manifests the all-pervading *Sabda-Brahman*."[14] This is the deepest, unmanifested state of sound. What follows is the state of the sound or of the already manifested but causal word, which is formless. This state corresponds to the area in the body between the chakra of the solar plexus and the chakra of the heart. What follows is the manifestation of sound on the plane of those forces that are both endowed with form and shaping reality. This manifestation corresponds to the area between the chakra of the heart and that of the larynx. From the larynx on, sounds and words assume an audible, spoken, human form and thus become concretely manifested. Usually a jiva recognizes a sound only when it reaches that last phase, and he believes that this alone is a word, the same way he believes that only the physical body is his real body. On the contrary, as the physical body implies the subtle and causal bodies, which are its roots, likewise, the spoken word implies the subtle, causal, and unmanifested states of the word, up to the elementary power (kundalini). Without all this, the spoken word itself would not be possible, and more specifically, it would have no correspondence with reality, since the correspondence between a name and an object, as well as the evocative power of the sensible word, would be based on states of sound in which the objective (*artha*) and the subjective (*shabda*) dimensions are encompassed in a wider unity. Otherwise, language would be like the muttering of a delirious or crazy person.

As in the case of the three seats of *atma* beyond the waking state, the deep dimensions of the word elude the consciousness of the common person, who pronounces words only through the larynx, and who evokes like a ghost, through a word deprived of its primordial power, shadows and echoes of names rather than true names. Thus the doctrine of mantras represents an organic part in the transcendent process of reintegration, which constitutes the main goal of Tantric sadhana.

Like every *devata* and every natural element, each individual has his own name and mantra, an essential and eternal name, which corresponds to his supertemporal being and which usually has no relation with his first or last name. It is the name of the god of which he is the manifestation. That the bestowal of a name, in the Catholic ceremony of baptism, acquires the dignity of a sacrament may constitute a pale reflection or image of an initiatory rite. In that rite, the name bestowed was not arbitrary, but somehow corresponded to a mantra, to the eternal name of the individual, and to one of those names that in Western tradition "are inscribed in the stars," or in the Tree of Life. In the East it often happens that a spiritual teacher may indicate to this or to that person their own names, which are as secret as their mantras. It may happen, however, that this name is known only in its dormant form, so that it remains unintelligible to its recepient. Sir John Woodroffe, who was an Englishman, recalled that somebody had naively gone to him to ask him to explain the meaning of the mantra that he had received from his guru as his initiatory and secret name several years before. This clearly shows us the origin of a superstition that is found among some primitive people. They are afraid to reveal their names to outsiders because they believe that if somebody learns their names, that person may enslave their soul. These represent degenerated reminders and echoes from a very distant past, in which the name had the value of a mantra.

According to the Tantras, the mantra, in its magical use, integrates *sadhana-shakti*, which is the power that the apprentice acquires through given disciplines, being endowed with a divine force that is the mantra's shakti. The effectiveness of the magical action is the result of the union between these two shaktis. The I, through the vivified and awakened mantra, comes in contact with the "seed" of a given power and unites with it in a way that makes the act effective, even on the plane of objective reality. By incorporating in a given command the mantra related to the force found in any given phenomenon—this is above all an inner act, since the verbal expression is only its vehicle—the command is realized in a supernatural way, without the condition brought about by the habitual physical determinisms. For instance, he who knows the mantra of fire, by awakening and pronouncing it, may at will produce the manifestation of fire, since he acts with the seed of fire, which is superior and prior to any particular combustion. The mantra offers a body of power to the individual will. The texts say that *jaiva-shakti* (the power of the individual) is exalted by *mantra-shakti* in a *daivi-shakti*, which is a divine power; thus, in the term *vajra-vak*, because of the living word, the term *vajra* could also mean "scepter." Moreover, some Western magical traditions taught that "spirits," "angels," and "elementals" must obey those who know their true names. In the Kabbala the initiate was called "Lord of the Name" (*bal scem*). It must be said that, also because of contingent factors, these Western formulations lack the completeness and the general metaphysical bases of their Hindu counterparts.[15]

The mantra has the value of one of sadhana's instruments; its power is obviously related to the power of other instruments, and it is defined, generally speaking, by the overall spiritual level that has been reached by the apprentice.

· IX ·

THE SECRET RITUAL
THE USE OF ORGIES:
INITIATORY SEXUAL MAGIC

In Hindu and Shaivist Tantrism, the term *panchatattva* designates the so-called secret ritual, which is reserved for the viras. The texts give great importance to this ritual, and they even claim that if *panchatattva* is not practiced in one way or another, the worship of Shakti is impossible.[1] Since *panchatattva* includes the use of intoxicating beverages and the participation of women, in India it has been branded orgiastic and immoral. Consequently, some Westerners have formulated a negative opinion of Tantrism. The employment of sex for initiatory, ecstatic, and magical purposes is not a prerogative of Hindu Tantrism alone, however. It is also found in Buddhist Tantrism, in Tantric trends within Vaishnavism, and in the so-called schools of Sahajiya and of the *natha-siddhas*. I will discuss separately the use of sex at a yogic level.

Panchatattva literally means five elements. Reference is made to "five substances to be employed." These substances have been associated to the five great elements in the following way. Sexual intercourse (*maithuna*) corresponds to ether; wine or inebriating drinks (*madya*) to air; meat (*mamsa*) to fire; fish (*matsya*) to water; some cereals (*mudra*) to earth.[2] Since the names of all five substances begin with the letter *m*, the secret Tantric ritual has also been called *panchamakara*, "the ritual of the five *m*s."

The ritual assumes various meanings according to the level at which it is performed. In its most exoteric version, which is practiced in the Way of the Right Hand, the ritual aims at implementing the sacralization of the natural functions of nutrition and sex. The basic idea is that the ritual is not supposed to be a sophisticated ceremony overlapping real life, but that, on the contrary, it should affect life and permeate even its most practical dimensions. Anything that the animalistic person (pashu) does in an obtuse way, being driven by the tamasic impulses of need and greed, must be performed by the vira with an open and liberated mind, as if it were a ritual or a cosmic offering.

All of this still does not have a specifically Tantric character. The sacralization and ritualization of life has been a characteristic of Hindu civilization as well as of any other traditional civilization, with the exception of some strict ascetic groups. There is also a Christian saying: "Eat and drink for the glory of God." The pre-Christian West knew sacrificial meals. The Roman *epulae* for a very long time had a religious and symbolic counterpart; in them there was a reflection of the ancient belief concerning the encounter between humankind and the gods.[3]

A difficulty may arise when, besides food, Tantrism advocates the inclusion of women and of intoxicating beverages. This difficulty may be felt only from the standpoint of the religion that became predominant in the West. This religion, Christianity, has been dominated by a sex phobia, and it has considered the sexual act impure and unfit to be sacralized. This negative attitude should be considered anomalous, however, considering that the sacralization of sex and the conception of the sexual *sacrum* were typical of several traditional civilizations. This conception, incidentally, is also to be found in India. It was a Vedic idea that sexual union could be elevated to the rank of *ieros gamos*, a sacred union and a religious act, and that in these terms it could even have a propitiating spiritual power.[4] In the Upanishads sexual union is represented as a sacrificial action (the woman and her sexual organ are the fire in which the sacrifice is burned). In them it is possible to find various formulas that propitiate the cosmic ritualization of a conscientiously performed intercourse (not of a merely lusty one), in which man relates to woman as Heaven to Earth.[5]

Even the tradition of sacred beverages and of ritual libations is very ancient and is found in several civilizations. As far as India is concerned, during the Vedic period *soma*, which is an intoxicating beverage derived from a bitter plant, played an important role. In the use of similar beverages, the ritual dimension should be distinguished from the initiatory and magical dimension.

Therefore, at this first level there is nothing extraordinary, at least from a Western point of view, in the so-called Tantric sexual ritual. In the West, in fact, it is quite normal to indulge in meat, sex, and liquor. In India the Tantric ritual is anomalous, however, since India is predominantly vegetarian and the use of intoxicating beverages is extremely restricted.

Let us now turn to the second level of *panchatattva*, in which subtle elements play a major role. On the one hand, a text presents the image of a seed sown into the crack of a rock, which cannot sprout and germinate.[6] In this sense, the vira enjoys the five substances (*panchatattva*) and absorbs and transforms the powers inherent to them. On the other hand, the possibilities offered by *panchatattva* are seen in relation to the correspondences of the five substances with the "five great elements" and even with the five *vayus* or *pranadis*, which are the currents of the vital breath (prana). Prana belongs to the plane of subtle forces and not to the plane of material and organic forces. Every organic function has as its counterpart a form of these forces. More specifically, whenever the organism ingests a given substance, a current of vital breath is activated. At that point, what takes place is a momentary surfacing or flashing of subtle forms of consciousness within the organic subconscious. Those who enjoy a high level of subtle sensibility, thanks to specific disciplines that I have previously described, will be able to notice these flashes and to enter into contact with the powers or "great elements" that correspond to the five substances. Experiences of this kind are facilitated by mental states in which the masses of psychic power enclosed in the body are activated through an adequate stimulation.

Usually the correspondences are presented in the following terms. Ether corresponds to women and to prana (prana understood as an absorbing force that descends from the nostrils down to the heart, and as a subtle and solar current). Air corresponds to intoxicating beverages and to apana, which is a current flowing downward from the heart, through an action that resists any unification process. Fire corresponds to meat and to *samana*, which is the current of organic assimilation, which operates by altering and by amalgamating. Water corresponds to fish and to *udana*, the fluid breath that regulates bodily discharges. Earth corresponds to starchy foods and to *vyana*, which is an incorporating current. When resorting to *panchatattva* at this second level, one should be able to detect and to differentiate these effects as well as the subtle modifications that are determined by the five substances. According to those who perform such practices, in the case of the participation of women, the dominating perception is the feeling of something that breaks off and becomes detached. In the case of intoxicating beverages one experiences the feeling of expanding and of disappearing into thin air. In the case of starchy foods, one has the feeling of being wounded. These are, for the most part, negative sensations that need to be transformed into active states.

It is well known that in the context of ascetic and initiatory disciplines, sexual abstinence is highly recommended, since sex is reputed to be an obstacle to spiritual development. Everything depends on one's attitude, however. The view of the Path of the Left Hand is well known: to transform the negative into positive. Usually, indulgence in sex and in alcohol carries dissipating consequences from a spiritual as well as from a psychological point of view. But if one is endowed with the principle of a pure and detached force (*virya*), the very same dissipating states can bring release, favor a process of self-transcendence, and reduce tamasic residues.

As far as eating meat (instead of following a vegetarian regimen) is concerned, this is a different story. The consumption of meat is discouraged from a spiritual standpoint because of the fear of "infections," since the assimilation of this kind of food by the human organism involves the assimilation of subtle and psychological elements found in the subhuman and animal dimensions. The danger can be avoided if one possesses a sensibility acute enough to be aware of these infections and of the presence of a "fire" powerful enough to transform and to absorb them. In that event, the activation of the animal and elementary substratum enables one to absorb a stronger power. This situation reminds us of the seed sown in the crack of a rock and of the general Tantric principle of transforming poisonous substances into vital energies, "into veins and arteries." This is probably why it has been claimed that the ritual use of intoxicating beverages, in the context of *panchatattva*, makes old people become young again; that consumption of meat improves one's mind, inner energy, and strength; and that the consumption of fish restores one's generative power.[7]

It is clear by now that *panchatattva* is a sacred ritual reserved for the viras, and that it should not be popularized or practiced by pashus (especially in regard to sex and alcohol). The same applies to the Buddhist and Hindu varieties of such a ritual.

119

As far as intoxicating beverages are concerned, I have already mentioned that their employment as sacred beverages dates back many centuries and is found in several traditions. I would like to emphasize the role that soma played in the Vedic tradition (*soma* is the equivalent of the Persian *haoma*). Soma has been considered as a "nectar of immortality" (*amrita*), a term that is etymologically identical to the Greek term *ambrosia*. Both terms literally mean "no death." The Vedas also mention an immaterial or heavenly soma.[8] According to one tradition, the knowledge and the use of the heavenly soma at one point was lost. In order to achieve ecstasy and states of "divine enthusiasm," (*mania*, in the platonic meaning of the term) humans needed the aid of the earthly soma, which is a beverage extracted from the bitter milkweed. In concomitance with a right inner motivation and attitude, the ensuing inebriation may generate ecstatic and even initiatory feelings, hence the sacredness attributed to this beverage. In Dionysian practices, wine performed a similar function. In ancient mystery literature, the expression "sacred orgy" is a technical expression, frequently employed.[9] In Persian mysticism wine and inebriation have a double meaning, both literal and symbolical. In the context of the tradition of the Templar Knights, Guenon has remarked that the expression "to drink like a Templar" may have had a secret and magical meaning, very different from the exoteric and popular meaning that eventually became predominant. Also, in Patañjali's Yoga-Sutra (4:1), the mention of the "simple" substances associated with samadhi may refer to the use of analogous auxiliary elements.

The employment of intoxicating beverages and of sexual orgies is also found in Tantrism. Wine is called, in this context, "causal water" (*karanavari*) and "water of wisdom" (*jnamrita*). In the Kularnava-Tantra it is written: "*Brahman's* form (*rupa*) is enclosed in the body. Wine can help to reveal it: this is why yogins use it. Those who use wine for their own selfish pleasure instead of seeking the knowledge of *brahman* are guilty of a serious offense, and are therefore damned."

Another Tantric text sees in these substances the "liquid form" of Shakti herself, who is believed to be a redeeming goddess (Dravamayitara = "Savior in Liquid Form"). In this form she bestows liberation and enjoyment of earthly goods and removes every sin. Wine "has always been drunk by those who have experienced the ultimate liberation, and by those who have either become initiated or who attempt to be initiated." At this level of *panchatattva*, intoxicating beverages should be drunk in view of liberation. Mortal beings who resort to them by dominating their instincts and by following Shiva's law (dharma) are regarded as gods, and as "immortals on earth."[10] Reference to the law of Shiva, who is the god of active transcendence, is significant in this context. On the one hand the apprentice is encouraged to drink "until the sight or the mind is not affected."[11] On the other hand, in the Tantra there is a saying that has scandalized quite a few people: "One achieves liberation by drinking, by collapsing on the floor, and by getting up to drink some more." Some commentators have given an esoteric-symbolic interpretation to this saying, which, in their view, is related to kundalini yoga. According to these scholars, the saying refers not to intoxicating beverages but rather to further efforts that are necessary in order to lead the awakened kundalini higher and higher within one's body. As in many other cases, however, this saying can have more than one meaning, and it may even be taken literally. The apprentice should reach a certain level of intoxication and then reaffirm himself and overcome any collapse, all the while preserving the consciousness and the fundamental sense of the experience.

The ritual can have a collective dimension and thus resemble an orgy. It is performed in a circle or initiatory chain (chakra) of members of both sexes. In the ritual the use of wine is associated with the use of sex. In this context, though, those lascivious aspects that are usually evoked by the word orgy are mitigated by the presence of specific ritual procedures. It does not matter what the intoxicating beverage is extracted from (Indian wine is not made with grapes), but it is an essential requirement that the beverage be "purified" in order to produce the expected results.

"To drink wine that has not been purified is like drinking poison." Wine that has not been purified turns the kaulas into brutes: they should never partake of it. This impure wine does not produce any results and the devata—divinity or shakti—who resides in it is not propitiated. The preliminary purification may require a complex, contemplative, and ritual procedure, which is aimed at inducing a state of being in which the apprentice effectively establishes a contact with spiritual forces and acts in an ecstatic and sacred way. This is almost a process of transubstantiation, in which the magical imagination and various mantras are present. Two of these mantras are, for instance, HRIM (the mula-mantra of the primordial power) and PHAT ("the mantra of the sword"), which is often employed when the apprentice attempts to separate subtle elements from thick and material ones.

The preliminary stages of the purification are practiced in a circle (*chakra*) under the guidance of the "lord of the circle" (*chakrashvara*) who sits in the middle of the circle in front of the elements that must be purified. The *chakrashvara* then pronounces the traditional formula concerning the oneness of the person performing the sacrifice, of the sacrifice itself, and of the god the sacrifice is offered to. Then he draws at his left side, in a bright red color, a graphic symbol consisting of two intersecting triangles, which represent the metaphysical dyad (the god and the goddess), with either a circle (representing emptiness) or another inverted triangle inscribed in the hexagram. The second triangle, pointing downward, represents Parashakti. It is the equivalent of the metaphysical emptiness and represents transcendence, which is beyond the divine dyad. A ritual vessel (*kalasha*) containing the intoxicating beverage is put on the hexagram. The lord of the circle then evokes the presence of the goddess in himself and in the beverage with the help of the magical imagination. Ritual formulas are employed. The most important visualization aimed at directing the process is that which evokes the vital principle (*hamsah*) in the form of a solar force radiating "in the middle of a pure sky" or in the form of a force residing in the intermediate region, located, just like air, between heaven and earth. This causes the operation to shift from a physical to a metaphysical plane. An important aspect in the purification process is the ritual of the covering, which is associated with a specific gesture. The vessel is covered with a veil to signify that the material beverage covers the sacred beverage. In the course of the ritual, the veil covering the goddess who is asleep in the beverage (Devi Sudha) is removed, and the wine in the vessel thus becomes a "heavenly drink" (*divya-sudha*). The goddess is also referred to as Amrita (ambrosia, or deathless element). The purification process is completed with the uplifting of the curse associated with such beverages. This curse is believed to have been cast on intoxicating beverages by Brahma because of the evil deeds that they tend to promote.[12] We may conclude that this, rather than an allegory, is a ritual neutralization of the negative effects resulting from the consumption of this kind of beverage. Finally, the lord of the circle imagines the god and the goddess having intercourse inside the intoxicating beverage, which gradually becomes saturated with the deathless element. All of this creates the inner and subtle conditions necessary for a spiritually fruitful consumption of these beverages. The efficacy of the ritual is increased by the fluid vortex that is fed by the couples surrounding the *chakrashvara* as they evoke the same images and as they perform the same spiritual actions. It is said that the role of the lord of the circle may be played only by one who has been fully initiated.[13] He alone can direct the ritual and distribute the beverage. Once these requirements are fulfilled, the initiatory chain or circle is believed to be divine. Only those "who are pure of heart, who are unaffected by the external world, who see no differences, but to whom all things are the same, and who have realized the *brahman*,"[14] may become part of this chain. The Rudrayamala even says that wine should be drunk exclusively during the ritual.

What has been said so far should make it clear that *panchatattva* is not an orgy in the popular and profane sense of the word, even though it is possible to encounter degenerated and dissolute versions of it.

MAITHUNA

Having described the role that beverages play in *panchatattva*, let us now examine the role of sacred sexual intercourse (*maithuna*), which has been associated with the element ether. It is important to distinguish several planes or levels in *maithuna*.

First, it is possible to detect some residues of obscure practices that are derived from sorcery rather than from magic. This is the case, for instance, of those rituals in which a man, in order to achieve certain powers (siddhis), attempts to capture female entities (*yakshini* or *dakini*). The apprentice seduces and subdues these entities by casting a spell on a real woman and by possessing this real woman in a deserted place, such as a forest or a cemetery. It must be noted, however, that the pattern of these obscure practices is analogous to that of initiatory practices, so much so that the latter could be considered an elevation of the former onto a higher plane. Conversely, the obscure rituals may be considered a degenerated or demonic facsimile of the initiatory practices.

Second, it is important to acknowledge the role of collective orgiastic ceremonies. Some people saw in these practices the survival or the continuation of seasonal fertility rites. It is well known that the agrarian and seasonal interpretation of various ceremonies is an obsession of ethnologists and of some historians of religion. The main and basic purpose of the practice of orgies is a wild deconditioning of one's being. Some obscure forms of ecstasy are realized through promiscuity, the temporary removal of all inhibitions, and the revocation or orgiastic reenactment of the primordial chaos.

It should be noted that some orgiastic collective ceremonies practiced in Tantrism promote depersonalization and the complete abrogation of all moral taboos. In fact, besides those orgies in which men choose their sexual partners, there are other kinds of orgies in which no personal choice is allowed, and in which the sexual partner is assigned at random. Women "put their jackets in a heap"; each man gets his companion by lot by selecting a jacket out of the heap of the shaktis' garments. His shakti is the woman to whom the jacket belongs.[15] If the woman is one's daughter or sister, the rules are not changed and one is supposed to go on with the ritual. In Tantrism one may find the ritualization of sexual orgies to parallel the ritualization of intoxicating beverages. These are rituals practiced by a circle (*chakra* or *rasamandala* = "the circle of intoxication or of frenzied emotions") made up of couples. A true vira is exempt from the rule, which applies to lower-level members, prescribing the use of one's wife, and thus he can use any woman he pleases. "Shiva's marriage" is also allowed in this context. This is a temporary union (Shiva is the "patron saint" of all that is out of the norm) with a young woman, which has to be consummated inside the chakra. This union, although not sanctioned by the traditional Hindu marriage ceremony, can be repeated several times. Only pashus are excluded from this practice, no matter what caste they belong to. The ritualization of an orgy is also guaranteed by the number of couples participating in it (fifty). Fifty is the number of the letters in the Sanskrit alphabet, which correspond to as many cosmic powers. The couples form a circle and "the lord of the circle"(*chakrasvara*) and his partner sit in the middle of it. It is also a symbolic and highly ritualistic fact that while all women are scantily dressed, only the lord of the circle's partner is totally naked. As every woman represents Shakti or prakriti, the naked woman is the image of Shakti or of prakriti free of forms, at an elemental level.

Unfortunately we do not possess any text outlining the development of the orgiastic ceremony. As in the case of intoxicating beverages, we may suppose the creation of a magical-ecstatic atmosphere and of some kind of fluid vortex originating from the couple sitting in the middle of the circle. This assumption may be warranted by the fact that *chakras* of this kind are summoned for practical purposes, for instance, to propitiate the good outcome of a king's military expedition. In this case the ritual orgy is performed in order to generate a spiritual state that will render the magical action efficacious.

Since the aim of the orgy is an immanent and spiritual one, the rules that apply to collective sexual orgies of *panchatattva* are the same that apply to the sexual intercourse of a single couple. Every man embodies the Shiva principle (purusha), while every woman embodies the Shakti principle (prakriti). During the ritual the man and the woman are supposed to identify, respectively, with their corresponding spiritual principles. Their union reproduces the union of the divine couple. The two principles (which in the manifested and conditioned world appear to be separated according to a dualism, the main expression of which is the male/female dyad) are temporarily represented, thus evoking the "androgynous Shiva" (Ardhanarishvara) and the oneness of the principle. From an experiential point of view, the sexual union experienced in this way has a liberating power that abrogates the laws of duality, generates an ecstatic feeling, and leads, at least temporarily, beyond the limits of the individual and samsaric consciousness. Man and woman become one with their respective ontological principles (Shiva and Devi), which are present in their being and in their body. Since the dualistic law is suspended, *samata*, the state of "identity" and of transcendence also known as *sahaja*, can be obtained during what is commonly referred to as *samarasa* (the simultaneous erotic rapture and consequent orgasm that unite two beings during intercourse). In other words, a special form of exalted and transfigured pleasure may be experienced, which is the foreshadow of *sambhodi* itself, namely, the absolute radical enlightenment and the achievement of the unconditioned *sahaja*. The Kularnava-Tantra even claims that the supreme union can be achieved only through sexual intercourse.

This individual practice obviously grants results that are spiritually far more effective than those achieved in an orgy. Sexual experiences of an ecstatic type should be distinguished from those of a properly initiatory and yogic type, in which the sexual union is performed after a due process is observed. The yogin first applies a specific technique and emphasizes the ritualization and the evocation process. This is what characterizes the further level in the Tantric participation of women.

Let us now examine some interesting details. First of all, the young woman participating in the *panchatattva* and in similar rituals is called, besides shakti, *rati*. This word means "the beginning of *rasa*." *Rasa*, in turn, means rapture, intense emotion, and even orgasm. It should be noted that ancient Hindu tradition associated the state of intoxication with the Great Goddess in one of her forms, that of Varunani. In the Pali language though, *varuni* designates an intoxicating beverage and even an intoxicating woman. There is no doubt concerning the relationship between *varuni* and intoxicating beverages, since in some texts the expression "to drink Devi Varuni" refers to the consumption of such drinks. Even in the hymns of the strict ascetic Shankara, the goddess is associated with them, by virtue of being described as holding a cup or as being drunk. In this archetype or divine image the woman is perceived as the embodiment of rapture and of intoxication, so much so that her presence is related to the use of intoxicating beverages in the secret ritual of the Path of the Left Hand. In conclusion, the name *rati* ascribed to the vira's sexual partner designates one "whose essence is intoxication."

The Sahajiya school has elaborated an almost scholastic classification of various *ratis*, and it has indicated *vishesha-rati* as an exception and as the most proper type for initiatory practices. "Ordinary" women (*samanya-rati*) and "lustful" women (*sadharani-rati*) should be excluded from the ritual. On an initiatory level, it is said that while a vira belonging to the lower grades of the hierarchy should avail himself only of his spouse, this restriction does not apply to a true siddha, who is free to join with any woman in the course of the ritual, without restriction of caste. The texts of Vajrayana and of Tantric Vaishnavism describe the vira's partner as a type of woman that most Westerners would characterize as "dissolute." In truth, this is no longer the traditional marriage ceremony typical of the higher Aryan castes, but rather a technical magical and yogic operation in which the woman is valued not for her own individual qualities but only insofar as she represents an elemental force and some sort of fluid to be used in a process of spiritual "combustion." Tantric Vaishnavism sanctions this irregular union since (1) the divine couple, which a man and a woman should represent in their union, is that of Krishna and Radha, a couple violating the conjugal bond, and (2) the "ideal" and intense love is not the love existing between a married couple, but rather is *parakya* love, which is love for a young girl.[16]

Some texts consider various degrees of a woman's nudity. In the collective rituals only the lord of the circle's partner is stark naked. This is allowed only for the viras of higher levels. The ritualistic-symbolic implications of these norms are obvious: a woman's nudity evokes the naked, elementary state of Shakti, whom she incarnates. At a higher level, in which magical evocations are employed together with ritualism and symbolism, physical nakedness symbolizes a woman devoid of her own individuality, and of her human and personal characteristics. This woman becomes the embodiment of the "absolute woman," and of a power that may be so dangerous that only those who have a special Shaivist spiritual qualification can truly partake of her without incurring any serious consequence. An alchemical-Hermetic saying goes: "Happy are the Actaeons who can see the naked Diana and not die," in reference to the invulnerable and deadly Diana.[17]

At the level of individual initiatory exercises, it is said that a young woman must be consecrated prior to her participation, and initiated and instructed in the art of mudras, the magical and ritualistic positions. These women, besides *rati* and shakti, are sometimes referred to as *mudra*, a word that designates the yogic ritual positions that induce a given fluid state. The term designates the young woman in reference not only to the positions that she will assume during lovemaking but also to the evocation of a power within her, which assimilates her to a magical form of a divinity or to a divine attribute. Another designation for the woman is *lata*, which means "climbing plant." The term alludes to a position in which the woman clings to the man as he is sitting still, thus playing the active role in the sacred intercourse (*viparita maithuna*). The texts often refer to a preliminary phase based on the visualization of the asana (ritual postures) of the divine couple Shiva and Shakti. The woman must be loved "according to the ritual." She must first be worshiped (*puja*) and then possessed and enjoyed (*bhoga*). The meaning of worship varies according to the Tantric levels at which it is practiced. On an initiatory and magical level, it corresponds to the already-mentioned animation and projection of an image through the magical imagination, until the *devata* is evoked and invited into the flesh and blood of the young woman. To designate this procedure, the technical term *aropa* is employed, which means "bestowal of a different nature" onto an object, while its form and sensible appearances (*rupa*) remain the same. In this case what takes place is a temporary transubstantiation of the woman, which gives rise in her to a "real presence," or to the "absolute woman." *Aropa* is considered a necessary condition.

Another term designating women engaged in Tantric sexual practices, besides *rati, shakti, mudra,* and *lata,* is *vidya,* a word that means "knowledge," "wisdom," not in an abstract and intellectual sense, but in the sense of an awakening and transfiguring power. This is related to an aspect of femininity to which one may associate the allusions, found in some texts, to woman as guru, to the "initiating woman," to the "*vajra's* mother," or to the "origin of transcendent knowledge." We should not exclude the likelihood that such allusions relate to a matriarchical area (especially when the superiority of an initiation bestowed by a woman is upheld), to those "women's mysteries" that are found even in the ancient West, and which are not without relation to the sacred prostitution exercised in the name of a female deity, the Great Goddess. In this context, man participates in the *sacrum* only through woman and through intercourse with her. It is legitimate to think that all of this is closely associated to Tantrism, and that in a Tantric context Shiva (whose principle is represented by man) is incapable of action unless he is vivified by Shakti. Thus, the yogini, the vira's partner, is credited with the power to "free the essence of the I." In a Vishvasara-Tantra hymn it said that Durga "confers buddhi," *buddhi* meaning the transcendent intellect. From another point of view, the woman is potentially endowed with this principle, which she unleashes together with the inebriation and feeling of ecstasy induced by it. Thus in Buddhist Tantras, in which *prajna* has the same meaning of *vidya*, we find unorthodox buddhas who achieve enlightenment through intercourse with a young woman. On the metaphysical plane, these Tantras indicate as the supreme state the so-called *mahasukhakaya*, which is beyond mere nirvana. On this plane, Buddha is embraced by Shakti, or by Tara. Only on this plane do the buddhas enjoy full possession of *buddhatva*, thanks to the ecstasy, of which she is the source, and to the creating power, of which she is the origin. In Vajrayana spiritual realization requires the union, symbolically represented as an embrace, of prajna and *upaya*, that is, of the illuminating knowledge (female principle) and of the operating power (male principle). The symbol, in turn, is turned into reality: woman embodies prajna, and man *upaya*, and their sexual union is called *vajrapadmasamskara* (*samskara* = action, sacrament, or magical operation; *vajra* and *padma* designate the male and female sexual organs).

This distribution of the masculine and feminine roles appears to exclude a matriarchical initiation, or an initiation in which the female principle is predominant. The woman is almost a mother figure ("the womb of the *vajra*"), since she generates the excitement and the ecstasy that vivify and enlighten the I principle of the man, who is the potential bearer of the diamond-thunderbolt (*vajra*). But this mother is also the woman with whom the man commits "incest," in the context of a union in which the moment of the *vajra's* birth and awakening coincides with the moment of the shakti's penetration and absorption. We may assume, therefore, that from an inner point of view the embrace consists of two phases, the meaning of which is best expressed by European alchemical Hermetism. Hermetists employ the symbol of the lunar female who prevails over the solar male, absorbs him, and makes him disappear within herself. Eventually the male asserts himself, mounts the woman, and reduces her to his own nature. This is symbolized by the mother's generating the son and by the son generating, in turn, the mother. In Tantric terms, this means that Shakti assumes Shiva's form, and that she becomes *chidrupini-shakti*. I previously discussed this transformation on a cosmological plane, as the meaning of the second phase of the manifestation (the ascending phase). Under this particular aspect, the vira's mate is purely Shaktic; she is the "absolute woman" led by an elementary desire. She is animated by the same force yearning for the *vajra-sattva*, the male principle that quiets her, soothes her tension, and bathes her in the cold, pure light of the magical one.

For the Tantric practice to be efficacious, it must awaken the pure Shaktic quality in femininity and act as something dangerous and destructive, for this is the essence of the Path of the Left Hand, namely, to seek out dissolving, "toxic" situations and to find in them liberation as the final outcome. Precisely because of the woman's characteristics and because of the nature of the states that arise during intercourse with her, it is a categorical necessity for those who follow the pure ascetic and contemplative path to stay away from her.[18] On the other hand, when it is necessary that the young woman, besides her natural qualifications, be initiated and adequately trained, it is likely that this training will extend to the art of physical love and to its magical counterparts. At a yogic level, as we shall learn later on, the young woman is required to have a special control of the vaginal muscles. Those who are familiar with the erotic Hindu treatises know that they suggest erotic positions that European women would not even consider, because they require a very difficult physical training.

That the vira should not lose control of himself during the sexual experience, and that the interpretation of such an experience in terms of the two phases alluded by the Hermetic-alchemical symbolism is truly adequate, is beyond any doubt. Generally speaking, there are precepts concerning the purification of the will: "Dominating his senses, detached, impassible when confronted by pairs of opposites, steady in the principle of his own strength," the vira practices *panchatattva*. The Kularnava-Tantra repeats that he must be well determined in his mind and will, and that his senses must be purified and mastered. Another text specifies that this self-control should be maintained throughout all the stages of passion (*rasa*) that arise during intercourse. The congenital tendency in the pashu to lose himself in physical pleasure and to give in to any desire of the flesh must be neutralized; in all likelihood the expression "purity of the senses" should be understood in these terms. Vajrayana texts warn against the abuse of sexual practices and call "two-legged beasts" those who are guilty of such abuses, and who therefore should not be mistaken for true viras.

There is also a significant precept prohibiting the vira to subject himself to hypnotic experiments. It is possible that the texts envisioned the danger of the vira becoming subject to a deleterious fascination during the encounter with the shakti-woman, and to a subsequent fall. It is also said that the body must be in perfect shape and strengthened through the use of hatha yoga, lest the crucial experience turn into fainting or swooning: "Without a perfect body, the *sahaja* cannot realize himself."

In relation to the principle according to which self-control must be exercised in all of the phases of sexual intercourse, sometimes a corresponding preliminary discipline is considered. In a ritual of the Sahajiya school, a man must spend time with the young woman he wishes to possess, and sleep where she sleeps, without touching her, on a separate bed, for a period of four months. After that, he should sleep next to her, on her left side, for another four months, and for four months on her right side, all this time without ever touching her. Only after this ordeal is he allowed to initiate the magical intercourse with the naked woman, thus beginning the operative phase. There are other, simplified forms of an analogous preliminary discipline. Their goal certainly does not consist in developing a sense of familiarity, which would weaken the desire. It should not be left out that this ritual has two phases, the first one consisting in a "subtle" intercourse without physical contact ("platonic"), the woman-goddess being the object of adoration. The second phase would be considered the extension of the first, in which the union is consummated on the physical plane as well, "in conformity to the ritual," which presupposes it. Such a supposition is plausible if we consider that these two phases are considered in some of the teachings of sexual magic as it is taught nowadays in the Western world. In any event, the preliminary exercise of one's self-control by lying next to the woman seems to have a specific meaning also when we consider the character of the technique to be employed at a yogic level in order to prevent the usual outcome of average sexual intercourse.

Let us now focus on this last level, which is part of hatha yoga. It is not easy to gather details from the texts, because they typically employ a cryptic language. Therefore, the same terms have at times a symbolical meaning, referring to ontological principles and to spiritual operations, and at other times they have a concrete and operative meaning, referring to organs, bodily substances, physical actions. *Bindu*, for instance, the "dot," a term we came across when dealing with Tantric metaphysics, may also signify male semen, or sperm. *Vajra* may signify the male sexual organ, and *rajas* the female vaginal secretions. *Mudra* may signify the woman and *padma* her sexual organ, also called *yoni*. One meaning does not exclude the other, not only because they refer to different planes, but also because the spiritual meanings or elements may represent the counterpart of material and even physiological procedures or elements, since every operation takes place on a double plane, physiological and transphysiological, at the same time.

One thing is still not very clear. In hatha yoga sexual intercourse is considered a means to bring about a traumatic shift in the level of consciousness, as well as an effective opening to transcendence, but only when the intercourse is performed according to specific rules. These rules essentially prescribe the inhibition of the man's ejaculation and the release of even the smallest quantity of semen inside the woman's body. The semen should never be released. In this context, orgasm is seen as separated from its physiological conditions; its peak, which in man culminates with ejaculation, is transformed and thus occasions the intuition that overcomes the limits of ordinary, finite consciousness and that leads to the realization of the One. Some texts, such as the Hatha-Yoga-Pradipika also mention some auxiliary procedures, such as suspension of breath in its radical form (*khecari-mudra*, *mudra* here meaning "gesture-seal" rather than "woman"). By practicing *khecari-mudra*, it is said, "He cannot be aroused by the most passionate embrace, even if he were in the hands of an ecstatic lover."[19] Mention is made of a special type of mudra—*vajroli-mudra* or *yoni-mudra*. One, however, should not be deceived by the literal interpretation of the texts, according to which the procedure being discussed appears to be a merely physiological one. It is said: "Even when the fluid has been released into the female sexual organ, he [the yogin] can make it reascend to its source through the *yoni-mudra*." And also: "The yogin who can withhold his semen overcomes death. Just as the release of *bindu* leads to death, likewise its withholding leads to life."[20]

A woman properly trained in erotic techniques could help the yogin by compressing the male organ with her vaginal muscles right before ejaculation occurs. However, it is not easy to imagine how that is possible. Considering the tumescence of the male organ (*lingam*), even if a woman was endowed with highly developed vaginal muscles, it is unlikely that her initiative would be effective. On the contrary, it is most likely to produce the opposite effects, since usually this kind of pressure increases the man's excitement, thus making ejaculation irrepressible.

It seems to me that this technique may be best understood when seen in the light of other texts. In other texts, the inhibition of ejaculation is related to both the attainment of the *bindu-siddhi,* or of the energy contained in the *bindu,* and to the occult doctrine of the deathless element, or ambrosia. This deathless element is believed to descend from the middle of the forehead, and to be consumed and burned under the species of semen: hence the corruptibility of the human organism. This is not a mechanical procedure consisting in withholding a physical substance and in directing its movement inside the physical organs. It is rather an inner action that has as its object the force that "precipitates" and degenerates into semen. The purpose of this action is to suspend such a precipitation, and to induce this force to act on a different, or better, on a transphysiological plane. Thus it can be understood that the aforesaid mudra of the suspension of breath may be of great help, especially at the peak of intercourse, when all the material and emotional conditions for the precipitation of *bindu* and for ejaculation are present. After all, this interpretation is supported by the indications concerning yet another mudra, the *amaroli-mudra,* which is the woman's equivalent to the man's *vajroli-mudra.* The woman is required to operate an analogous suspension and retention of fluid, the designation of which is difficult to assess.

We should consider two factors in reference to the nonemission of semen. The first factor is that in the context of ordinary sexual love, and in some cases when an intense desire for a woman is present, the result may be absence of ejaculation. The second factor is that all the evocative processes provoke a natural shift of consciousness onto the subtle plane, which occurs in some sort of trance. This shift, in turn, causes the separation of vital energies from the physical and physiological plane; this may prevent ejaculation. Incidentally, the inability to achieve ejaculation is also found in the case of the consumption of drugs, since their use provokes, though in a passive way, the shift of consciousness onto the subtle plane. Even without the aforesaid yogic procedures, these two factors cannot but facilitate the fundamental operation of *vajroli-mudra*.

Once the precipitation of the semen-*bindu* is arrested, what usually corresponds to the fleeting peak of the orgasmic crisis is also stabilized in an exalted and transfigured form, or in a state of active trance. The texts speak of an "endless union," namely, of a state that lasts for a long time. Reference is made to an analogous theory concerning fire and the other elements. As there is an ungenerated and eternal fire that manifests itself in various combustion processes, likewise there is an ungenerated concupiscence, which corresponds to that which is expressed in the union of the divine couple Shiva and Shakti. The passion experienced by men and women during their mating is merely a pale, temporary, and contingent reflection of the divine concupiscence. It is assumed that a magical intercourse, when performed according to the aforesaid conditions, activates, attracts, and fixes such a pleasure in a transcendent form, which is "without beginning or end": hence the occurrence of an orgasmic peak that lasts, instead of the fainting feeling that men and women usually experience after the fleeting orgasmic crisis.

Thus, in the state called *samarasa* ("identity of pleasure," or unitive ecstasy, representing the fusion and dissolutive absorption of the male principle into the shakti employed), the goal at a yogic level is to experience the "thunderbolt" element, or that which is primordial, "ungenerated," or "unconditioned." The term for "ungenerated," *sahaja*, which has come to designate a Tantric school, has been used by Kanha (a late Madhyamika Buddhist school) as synonymous with "emptiness" or "transcendence." The texts talk about "immobilizing the king of the spirit through the identity of pleasure in the ungenerated state," which has as a consequence the immediate attainment of the principle at the basis of all kinds of magic, namely, the overcoming of time and of death. The sexual union crosses into the union of *padma* (which symbolizes the enlightening knowledge as well as the female organ and secretions) and *vajra* (which is the active spiritual principle as well as the male organ) with the result of producing the state of emptiness.

A Kabbalist-Hermetic text, the *Asch mezareph* (5), indicates the essential procedure through an esoteric interpretation of the biblical episode of Phineas's spear thrust, who "pierced *in locis genitalibus* the solar Israelite man and the lunar Midianite woman as they were having sexual intercourse. The sharpness and the strength of iron, by acting on matter, purifies it from all impurities. . . . Phineas's spear not only slays the male Sulphur but it also kills his female. And so they die, mixing their blood in the same one generation. Then Phineas's wonders begin."[21]

In this cryptic passage, taken from a Jewish source, we may gather an analogous teaching at an initiatory level concerning sexual magic. Significantly, it is said that in such practices one has to experience death in order to reach life; we may recall that orgasm is poetically referred to as "sweet death." The association of love and death is a famous theme found in several traditions and even in literature. This theme, if we go beyond the limits of a stereotypical and decadent romanticism, may be transferred onto an objective, operative plane. What is important is to activate fully that dimension of transcendence that is also hidden in all forms of intense profane sexual love.[22] Unlike the pashu, the ordinary man, who undergoes pleasure and experiences the surfacing of that transcendence as a spasm that impairs, dominates, and dissolves his inner being, the initiated person is supremely active and brings about some sort of enlightening short circuit. The stopping of the seminal flow, especially in unison with the suspension of breath, "slays the manas." What ensues is a state of active trance through a flow that "travels upstream," beyond this conditioned human existence. To know this procedure is considered the essential thing.

As an example of coded expositions, I will quote from Shahidullah's commentary to Kanha and to the Doha-Kosha:

> The supreme and most exalted enjoyment (paramahasukha) consists in the suppression of thought, in order that thought may become nonthought, in the state of the ungenerated. When breath and thought converge in the unity of enjoyment (samarasa) one achieves the supreme, great joy, and true annihilation. The joy consisting in the I's annihilation may be achieved during sexual intercourse, in the state of identity of enjoyment, when shakra and rajas are immobilized.

According to these teachings, the ritual that employs sex provokes, just as in hatha yoga, the suspension of the two currents ida and pingala, more on which later, as well as the ascent of the vital force through the sushumna. This exercise should be practiced only in the middle of the night, because of analogical and subtle reasons.

Mantras and images, too, seem to play a role in the development of the operation. The mantra that is found in the Hindu texts is Kali's own mantra, KRIM. Obviously, it is believed to have been awakened, at least partially. The basic image associated with it, in the course of practice, is that of the goddess who manifests herself in *rati* and who *is* this *rati*. The details of such an image resemble cult figures, and they are such that their suggestive and exciting power is strictly connected to the entire Hindu or Tibetan tradition. The image of Kali naked, surrounded by flames, her hair loose, wearing a necklace of severed heads, and dancing on the still body of Shiva, probably evokes a passionate and unleashed attitude. Some details can be found in a text called the Prapankasara-Tantra (28:27ff); in this text it is said that a woman must be realized as fire. In the following phases of the experience, a reference is made to a fire that, once the combustible material has been consumed, changes into a subtle state, free of all manifested forms. Then Shakti embraces Shiva and becomes one thing with him: this corresponds to the man's breaking point, to the transformation and to the growth into a timeless dimension of the sexual and orgasmic climax, which is caused by the ejaculation into the woman.

Considering the constant and faithful bearing of the symbolic, ritualistic, and metaphysical structures on the human and concrete plane, it is easy to understand why *viparita-maithuna* is chosen for the aforesaid yogic sexual practices. As I have indicated, this type of sexual intercourse is characterized by the woman wrapping her legs around the man and performing the acts of love on him as he sits still (the ritualistic stillness is the symbol of Shiva's unchanging nature).

Let us now consider the sexual experience from the woman's point of view. In the case of a collective orgy, whether of a promiscuous or of a ritualistic type, the level of participation of men and women is about the same. What women are supposed to do at a yogic level is not very clear because of the obscure language employed by the texts. Some texts seem to consider a special mudra (in the sense of an operation or gesture) for women, namely, the so-called *amaroli-mudra*, which is the counterpart of the *vajroli-mudra*, designating the suspension of ejaculation. In the Sahajiya texts the stopping and the immobilization are referred both to the male (*shukra*) and to the female "semen," and the two operations must occur simultaneously, in both man and woman, with the rising of the orgasmic tide. It is not clear what is meant by female semen. Mention is made of the "woman's *rajas*," but *rajas* has various meanings, among them "menstrual blood" and "vaginal secretions." Menstruation is out of the question, and it is also unlikely that when the texts refer to a woman's retention or immobilization of fluid they are actually referring to vaginal secretions. These secretions, in fact, are usually produced at an early stage of a woman's excitement, and sometimes they are even lacking. It is also unlikely that the texts refer to the woman's ovum, which does not descend into the woman's uterus when orgasm occurs. Thus we are left with an interpretation that is neither physiological or material: the woman's "semen" is a force that must be stopped before it degenerates into orgasm and into mere physical pleasure. This interpretation, besides explaining an otherwise unintelligible *amaroli-mudra* in the woman, confirms the analogous interpretation given to *vajroli-mudra*, the suspension of man's semen. In any event, it is clear that a woman's initiative is not supposed to jeopardize what I have called her "potentiality for combustion," which is her main part. It could not be otherwise, considering that during the intercourse the vira, after suspending his semen, absorbs the woman's *rajas*, which it caused to flow, and is nourished by it.[23] The woman's *rajas* is therefore present as a fluid or magical force that feeds the development of the *samarasa* state. This state would probably be affected if the woman withdrew from the intercourse or if she suddenly gave in to orgasm.

Let me now mention an unusual sexual practice found in Tantric Buddhism, whose purpose is regeneration in an almost literal and physical sense. This practice is called *mahayoga* or *mahasadhana*. It is difficult to define the plane on which it takes place. In it, "realized" images seem to play the key role. The man must imagine to be dead to his present existence, and now, taking the form of some kind of fecundating semen, he must penetrate a "supernatural matrix" (*garbhadhatu*). In a preliminary exercise, which consists in contemplation or dhyana, he duly recalls the process leading to his human birth. Man evokes the so-called *antarabhava*, which, according to a Hindu view, must be present at conception in addition to the egg and sperm cells. At the same time he must visualize the *hieros gamos*, the sacred intercourse between a god and a goddess, and he must evoke in himself an intense yearning for the goddess Tara. When a man couples with and desires a woman, the *antarabhava* identifies with the future father and during orgasm enters into the woman, being carried inside the semen. In the same fashion, an analogous process is imagined. In this process, the *vajra*, or buddha principle, which is carried by the god coupling with Tara, takes the place of the *antarabhava*. This preliminary dhyana aims at creating the scenario for the sexual union that will ensue, and at evoking and at directing one's inner powers. This practice also contemplates the use of mantras and the vivification of the body of the young woman through a *nyasa*. What ensues are various dedication and confirmation rituals, on which I am not going to elaborate. This Tantric Buddhist practice appears to be very complex. Its core idea is that of a regression into the prenatal state and of a regeneration to be accomplished with the same forces that intervene in the circumstances affecting conception and physical birth. The apprentice attempts to enter into contact with these forces, and after successfully combining them with transforming images, he reenacts the procreative act, which is believed to generate transcendent and spiritual results. In this way one destroys one's birth by reenacting the drama that determined it, and by performing an act in which the samsaric *antarabhava* is substituted by a principle of a buddha or Shiva nature. In this act the divine woman, or Tara, is evoked and comes to life in the body of the earthly woman, which she takes over.

It is only in these terms that we can approximately identify what concerns the employment of sex, while trying to find our way in the maze of illusions, the cryptic language, and the cultural images and symbols of Tantrism. In the Tantric yoga of sex, the idea of arising and of assuming the forces of desire (in order to make them self-consuming, that is, to transform, or better, to destroy their original nature) finds its most classical expression. Thus the practice that uses and excites the elementary power of desire (sexuality) is associated with the myth of Shiva as a mountain ascetic who through his frontal eye turns into ashes Kama, the god of concupiscence. This is a mythologization of what corresponds to *vajroli-mudra*. In fact, it is said that when the apprentice awakens the force of desire and when he performs *japa* (the procedure that awakens mantras) with a naked young woman (shakti), he becomes the earthly slayer of the god of love (*smarahara*). According to some Shaivist texts, these practices have a cathartic power; through them the kaula becomes free from all faults and achieves *jivanmukti*, namely, liberation while alive.[24] Tantric apologetic works describe the kaula who is expert in the *panchatattva* as a being who subdues every human power, as one superior to any ruler, and as a diviner. According to Tantric Buddhism, Buddha was able to overcome Mara (= Smara), the god of this earth and of desire, and to acquire transcendent insights and magical powers, by virtue of having practiced Tantric rituals that employ women.

Unlike what is proper to the viras of the lower grades and to the promiscuous orgiastic experience of the chakras, it is possible that a yogic level the operation of sexual magic will acquire an exceptional character. The goal is the initiatory and almost traumatic opening of one's consciousness to the unconditioned. Once this is achieved through the participation of women, it is still possible to go beyond, either by abandoning the practice or by repeating it only in particular circumstances. Thus Vajrayana itself presents figures of siddhas who, after practicing the sexual ritual and after having obviously reaped the benefits, renounce women, prescribe sexual continence, and abide by an austere discipline. Some texts suggest that to think otherwise is to commit a fatal mistake. But even in other cases, what I have said concerning the preparation, concerning all of the conditions necessary to a successful practice, and concerning the dangers inherent to these practices rules out the possibility that the viras' doctrine is merely a pretext and a cover-up for indulging in libidinous and dissolute pleasures. It is quite another thing, though, to claim that those who are siddhas, those who have reached the end of the Way, may eventually employ any woman of their choice, since they are free to do as they please. They do not know interdictions, and it is even claimed that siddhas, rather than Brahmans, are able to make the best use of women. Obviously this applies to a different plane, that of the freedom enjoyed by the Tantric adept.

It is important to specify the role that the yoga of sex occupies in the general hierarchy of sadhana's varieties. Some texts' hints may induce the reader to conclude that it may even lead to the awakening of kundalini, which is the main goal of hatha yoga, and that the end results of both types of yoga are more or less the same. Such a correspondence refers only to special forms or cases, however. It is more probable that if the sexual practice, in its magical and initiatory aspect, provokes even partially kundalini's awakening, kundalini, unlike what happens in classical yoga, is not mastered and led through the various powers and elements of spiritual corporeity (chakras). Especially at the level of *panchatattva*, we are confronted with a spiritual exploit that attempts to achieve, in a sudden intuition, the meaning of transcendence (*sahaja*) through the apex of a Dionysian experience that is transfigured and magically strengthened. The criticism that may be made from the perspective of classical yoga is that this is a transient achievement.

Although sometimes the texts suggest that besides the vira, who is characterized by the rajas guna, even the divya, who is characterized by the sattva guna, may practice the *panchatattva*, the proper domain of the second type is that of hatha yoga in the strict sense of the term. Even in the higher levels of *panchatattva* there is always an outer influence: the experience cannot be achieved by an individual without recourse to some external factors, such as, in the case of the most radical practices, intoxicating beverages and the participation of women. On the level of pure hatha yoga this influence from the outside, or this external element, is eliminated. I have already quoted a saying of a divya: "What need do I have of any outer woman? I have an inner woman within myself."[25] Sadhana is realized with one's own means, through operations that take place within one's body.

· X ·

THE OCCULT CORPOREITY
The Serpent Power:
The Chakras

The Hindu Tantric hatha yoga is synonymous with kundalini yoga. Its equivalent in Tantric-Buddhism is *vajrarupa-guhya*, "the mystery of the diamond-thunderbolt body (*rupa*)." At this level, sadhana focuses on the body, which constitutes its foundation and the place in which all spiritual operations take place. The presupposition of this kind of yoga is the analogical-magical correspondence between the microcosm and the macrocosm. All the powers that are actively manifested in the world are also actively present in the body. In a general sense, this idea is expressed in the Tantras by the saying "That which appears without only so appears because it exists within."[1] The Nirvana-Tantra declares: "Truly, each body is this universe (*brahmananda*)." This corresponds to another saying: "Listen, o goddess [the text assumes Shiva is instructing Shakti]: wisdom is to be found within the body. If one really discovers it, he will become omniscient."[2]

Obviously, the object of consideration here is not the physical body but rather the entire corporeity, and more precisely, the human body, which is perceived as an instrument of superphysical forces. These forces operate in the physical body and sustain it. It is necessary at this point to refer to the theory of the three bodies—

140

material, subtle, and causal bodies—which are not three distinct entities but rather three dimensions of the same entity. I have already said that the three bodies correspond to the three seats of consciousness. The material body corresponds to ordinary waking consciousness, in which one experiences the world in a physical and phenomenical way. This is the seat proper to the ordinary I. The other two bodies, or better, the other two dimensions of corporeity, ordinarily cannot be perceived. This is because in common people's lives, the subtle plane corresponds to the dream state (*svapnasthana*), while the state that comes after that (the causal state) corresponds to the dreamless state or to deep sleep (*sushupta-sthana.*) A fourth state (*kathurta* or *turiya*), which is the unconditioned, is the equivalent of a state of catalepsy, or of apparent death. Therefore, the deeper, transphysiological dimensions of human corporeity are precluded to common men's waking consciousness. Neither can they experience the rajas state of corporeity as pure energy (subtle body), nor can they experience the sattva state as pure act (causal body), since both of those states are not limited to a single body. Ordinary men know and are subject to only the tamas state of corporeity. They live in what may be considered a particular, determined, static, and short-lived expression and manifestation of life, as if they were automatic "precipitates" in an exhausted process; this expression is the material body, *sthula-rupa*. The subconscious, the unconscious, and various forms of reduced consciousness (e.g., the dream state) contain and conceal the mystery of transcendent corporeity, and also block the access to it.

Hatha yoga techniques aim at removing this barrier and at revealing the spiritual corporeity to a clear and alert consciousness. This involves an expansion of consciousness itself, and its development into a superconsciousness that replaces those forms of impaired and dulled consciousness. I would like to suggest, at this point, that some absurd psychoanalytical interpretations of yoga are circulated in the West by people who are extremely ignorant of even the most basic principles of yoga. According to these interpretations, yoga is supposed to induce hypnotic or trancelike states (like those experienced by a medium) that are below, rather than above, the level of ordinary waking consciousness. Exactly the opposite happens to be true.[3] Western antiquity knew better, since Plutarch, for instance, wrote, "Not without divine inspiration has sleep spoken: it represents the lesser mysteries of death, since it is a preliminary initiation into death." Likewise, Synesius wrote, "Sleep discloses the path leading to a being's most complete fulfillment."

I think it is absurd to attempt to establish a connection between yoga and modern psychoanalysis, even if we exclude Freud's school and consider instead the pseudospiritual views of C. G. Jung. Psychoanalysis, as a matter of fact, operates on the mere plane of phenomenological psychology, and worse yet, it reifies or absolutizes the unconscious, presenting it as an impenetrable entity (Jung was very explicit about this). Therefore, according to psychoanalysis, the obstacle posited by an individual's consciousness is considered insurmountable. Various psychoanalytical schools can only speculate on what the content of the unconscious is all about, since they do not admit the possibility of a direct and an immediate knowledge of the unconscious. These schools have variously assumed the content of the unconscious to be the heredity of the species; or the experiences during infancy (Freud actually referred to the sexual life of primitive people); or the mental structures found mainly in the hallucinations of neuropathological patients (Jung did not hesitate to draw aberrant analogies between Eastern mandalas and the figures appearing in such hallucinations); or the so-called archetypes, which are transferred from a metaphysical plane to the plane of irrationality, of *bios*, of life, and, of the "entreaties" on the rational and social ego. The dimension under scrutiny is dark, materialistic, and merely physiological. In yoga, on the contrary, the unconscious incorporates ontological principles and metaphysical realities;[4] it may be resolved and known. In this case the unconscious gives way to a superconsciousness, and thus an authentic reintegration of the I takes place. Psychoanalysis reaches its most absurd conclusions when, in the person of Jung, it presumes to indicate the positive, "scientific" content of yoga and of related disciplines. Psychoanalysis claims that these Eastern disciplines merely attempt to heal neurotic and sick individuals who are plagued and torn by the conflicts and by the divisions between the conscious and the unconscious. Yoga does not purport to heal sick, neurotic, and tormented individuals, however. On the contrary, it presupposes a healthy, balanced person, to whom it will indicate the way to eventually overcome the human condition.

After this brief though necessary clarification, let us return to our subject. That the ordinary I's consciousness is somehow external to the body, since its seat cannot be physically located, is the reason why the world, too, appears to be external to the I. Thus, when one crosses the boundaries of ordinary consciousness and enters into the subtle and causal planes, what ensues is a different relationship with the world as well as the discovery of its nonphysical, nonphenomenological, or immaterial dimensions.

The state in which the I rests upon and is immersed into the occult corporeity corresponds to the individual's consciousness of having lived so far only once—that is, now, in this body. This is the natural consequence of the outwardness of ordinary consciousness vis-à-vis the forces acting deep down inside one's being; these forces, though they may be expressed in the physical body, are superior to every single individuation. We may speak here of "the dangers to the immortal soul," in the sense that physical death may not turn out to be an indifferent event after all but, on the contrary, may constitute a serious crisis. When the I is immersed and sunken into an individuated form, it participates, to a certain extent, in the finite and ephemeral nature of that form. This is not to say that when the bodily foundation of an individual's life is dissolved after the death of the organism, the force that became attached to and involved in the bodily foundation will just fade away. More properly, the continuity of consciousness has been broken. A real continuity is conceivable only at the subtle and causal bodies' level, since these seats are superior to every single individuation and production and are not limited to only one life.

At the level of the subtle body what surfaces is the "samsaric consciousness," or better, the awareness of being swept by a current in which a single existence merely represents a particular vortex. At the level of the causal body, consciousness extends vertically to multiple states of being, up to a point where there is no change or becoming. We may briefly recall that the East for a long time has known theories such as the theory of reincarnation, while more recently the West has professed almost exclusively the belief in the uniqueness of an individual's life. This fact, per se, is not a cause, but rather a consequence, or a barometric index, of the growing involution taking place during the dark age (Kali Yuga) to which I have often referred. Those Eastern theories still contain an echo of the primordial state in which ancient humanity once lived. In that state, the seat of the subtle body was not totally barred, and humanity still had a feeling of the "samsaric consciousness" connected to that seat. That knowledge was lost with the passing of time because the human body became increasingly physical. Naturally, as I have repeatedly stated, belief in reincarnation is folk-based and somewhat superstitious. Since this belief expounds the notion of a series of earthly incarnations of a single entity, it should be rejected as lacking solid, traditional foundations.

Let us return to hatha yoga. Its main requirement is the development of the doctrine of total corporeity in its macrocosmic correspondences, which are expressed in terms of an elaborate and occult anatomy and physiology. The basic teaching is that the elementary principles and forces active in the world (*bijas* and *devatas*) are present in the body in a series of centers that repeat the order of the manifestation, namely, the hierarchy of the tattvas. These centers—*chakras* (wheels) or *padmas* (lotuses)—are imperceptible, and they elude any research conducted with the means of modern experimental science. These centers emanate currents of vital and luminous force that relate to organic and psychophysical functions: hence the correspondence between physical organs or systems and "heavenly" powers (semipure tattvas) or "divine" powers (pure tattvas). I will discuss the chakras at greater length in the following pages.

There is a special relationship between organic systems and those states that characterize various bodies and seats of consciousness. According to yogic doctrine, these states, on a physical plane, have their corresponding "precipitates" in the cerebral system, nervous system, circulatory system, and skeletal system. These systems correspond respectively to the ordinary waking state, dream state, sleep state, and catalexis, or state of apparent death (*turiya*).

In those human forms in which it is possible to recognize the fundamental duality of Shiva and Shakti, Shiva represents the power that is the source of one's clear consciousness; conversely, Shakti represents prana, or vital breath, which envelops and permeates the entire organism as warmth does with water, oil with a sesame seed, fire with burning wood. The organism, therefore, appears to be interwoven with luminous forces and currents (*vayus* and *nadis*), which are constantly moving.

Besides the Shakti element, found in the Shiva-Shakti dyad, the primary power, Parashakti, is also present in the organism in the form of kundalini. Kundalini is the root of a being's deepest life. Its seat in the human body is the *muladhara-chakra*. *Muladhara* means foundation, or fundamental support. According to yogic occult physiology, the plexus of the *nadis* (luminous arteries in which the basic life force, which permeates and lives in the occult corporeity, flows), is located in the *muladhara-chakra*. This basic center also corresponds to the last of the principles of the manifestation, namely, to the earth's tattva (*prithivi-tattva*); the earth symbolizes the state of outward, sensory, and material experiences. In this center of the invisible corporeity, the power at the basis of every manifestation is asleep. The term *kundalini*, or *kundali*, literally means "wrapped up," and it conveys the idea of sleep, or of a latent and unutilized potential.

Kundalini's sleep has various meanings. The most conventional one is referred to the waking experience of a chaotic and dualistically minded world, in which the unity of power is not perceived. Thus it is said that samsara goes on and that we live in its snares for all the time kundalini is asleep.

I have briefly mentioned that there seems to be a relationship between kundalini and sex; thus magical-sexual practices are supposed to cause a temporary arousal of the force. This relationship exists only in the context of a superphysical physiology, in the sense that Shakti, who rescinds the ties of yearning in the human condition, also manifests herself in that condition in the form of yearning. This is said to be her samsaric and somewhat degenerated manifestation. In a highly symbolic Tantric icon Shakti is portrayed at the earth's level (the *muladhara-chakra*) as a snake wrapped around Shiva's phallus and resting its head on the phallus's orifice. We must refer to the metaphysical theory according to which animal or physical generation is an empty surrogate of spiritual generation.[5] The continuation of the species, through the use of sex perceived mainly as a generative power, represents a sort of ephemeral and earthly "eternity," or a facsimile of continuity, in the series of separated, mortal individuals that follow one another in time. This spatio-temporal continuity is a mere surrogate for the continuity that would be ensured by an ascending or vertical birth, or by a metaphysical integration that is well beyond the finite state of an individual who is conditioned by a specific physical body. Shiva's reproductive organ (phallus), is called *svayambhu-linga*, or "supportless" linga, since it has its principle within itself. The term alludes to the power proper to a different begetting, not physical, but transcendent and anagogic; a begetting into a perfect, unblemished, incorruptible, and eternal life. Kundalini's head is blocking the opening of Shiva's phallus, thus preventing the ejaculation of semen, which is the principle of such an endogenesis. This clearly signifies that polarization, in the sense of sexual desire and procreative energy, prevents the force of the Shaivist *svayam bhu-linga* from becoming explicit and from assuming its proper form. Thus it is clear that one of the fundamental presuppositions of hatha yoga is the change of polarity operated by that energy which manifests itself in the form of passionate and procreative sexuality.

At this yogic level, in which techniques aimed at obtaining a self-consuming arousal of the primordial force are no longer required, the precept of sexual abstinence, or chastity, assumes a specific, operative meaning. It is not possible, in the case of ordinary human beings, to subscribe to the orientation, or to the concupiscence of Shakti's manifestation, and at the same time to go on to awaken kundalini, which is Shakti's realization in its proper and pure form. The term *urdhavaretas*, which is found in some Tantric and hatha yoga texts, means "to flow upward," and it alludes to a change of polarity. This idea is evident even in the Gnostic symbolism of the waters of the great Jordan River, which, when flowing downward, give place to animalistic procreation within the "circle of generation" (samsara); when flowing upward, they generate gods and a "race without a king."[6]

In relation to kundalini's awakening, I find it necessary to add a few more notions of occult physiology that are pertinent to the forms in which the dual principle manifests itself and acts in the human organism. Hatha yoga pays special attention to the two subtle and vital currents (*vayus*). These are *prana* (in the specific sense of the general term), which is related to breathing; and *apana*, which is related to man's secreting and discharging functions, for instance, the ejaculation of semen. Even though they have an antagonistic character, the two currents are interconnected. Prana tends to flow upward and to become detached from the body; however, as a falcon tied to a rope is prevented from flying to its destination, likewise prana is held back by apana and vice versa. As a ball forcefully thrown on the ground bounces back, this is what prana does to apana, which is oriented downward:[7] hence an oscillation bearing ties with the existential restlessness and instability proper to finite beings, whose life, according to the Dhyanabindu-Upanishad, "is never steady." In some texts we find an interesting interpretation of the term *hatha* (as in *hatha yoga*). *Ha* is said to correspond to the prana current; *tha* to the apana current. The whole word (*ha* + *tha*) reveals the "secret of this type of yoga," namely, the unification of the two currents. A secret yogic procedure called *mulabhanda* consists in inverting the natural direction of the two currents, that is, in directing prana downward and apana upward. "Through *mulabhanda*, prana and apana, *nada* and *bindu* join together and the perfection of yoga is finally achieved." Obviously such practices presuppose mastery over the subtle currents of the organism, and for this purpose a teacher's (guru's) guidance is necessary.

More relevance is given in yoga to the dual correspondence of the subtle organism, which is found in the existence of two main opposite arteries called the *pingala* and the *ida*. The ida has a lunar character and corresponds to the moon; it is connected to the Shaktic principle. The pingala has a solar character and corresponds to the sun; is connected to the Shaivist principle. These arteries are believed to have colors, not in a real, physical sense, but rather in reference to the character of the psychic perception of various impressions. The ida is pale and ethereal, slightly pink, like the color of the almond flower. The pingala instead is bright red. They both depart from the *muladhara-chakra*, which is the chakra located where the sacrum joins the coccyx. They are intertwined like a spiraling serpent around the spine, touching five times along the axis of the spine, the last spot being at the level of the eyebrows, where, as in the portraits of various divinities, we find the so-called *urna*, the frontal stone that in Western mythology represents the Cyclops's eye and in Eastern mythology represents Shiva's third eye. They are believed to be related to the two lateral cords, left and right, that depend on the sympathetic nervous system, and also with alternating breathing from both nostrils (the yogins believe that we breath with one nostril and then with the other). The ida starts from the right testicle and terminates in the left nostril, while the pingala starts from the left testicle and terminates in the right nostril. According to the *hamsah* formulation of the vital principle (prana), the ida is associated with *sah*, or inspiration; the pingala, instead, is associated with *ham*, or expiration.

Interestingly enough, the duality of the ida and pingala is related to temporality (*kâla*), since the two currents measure the rhythm of the alternation of inspiration and expiration, which is typical of beings who live in time. Thus, when this duality is removed, because the pingala and ida are consumed in the one force that runs across the sushumna, time itself is consumed, and the temporal condition is suspended.[8]

The main way to light the fire that awakens kundalini consists in the suspension of the pingala's and ida's movement and in their conjunction. We might say that the conjunction of these two currents, one with a Shaivist-solar character, the other with a Shaktic-lunar character, acts as a sexual intercourse between man and woman (who represent respectively Shiva and Shakti). The suspension of the pingala and ida, obtained through pranayama, which is the control and suspension of the vital breath, arouses a fluid vortex that awakens kundalini. Once this elementary force is awakened, it absorbs and carries along with it all the other currents. It eventually goes beyond the barrier and ascends from the *muladhara-*

chakra along the spinal cord, around which, in ordinary life, the pingala and ida are intertwined. (The pattern of the three directions reproduces Hermes' caduceus, with two serpents wrapped around the central rod). The path along this axis is called the *sushumna*. What is usually called "*brahman's* threshold" (*brahmadvara*) is now crossed. This threshold is closed during the samsaric existential state, just as the opening of Shiva's phallus is symbolically closed in the *muladhara-chakra*. In its innermost part, the sushumna current is called *vajrini-nadi*, which signifies the nature of a diamond-thunderbolt. In even deeper recesses, it is called *chitrini-nadi*, since "it is radiating with the splendor of the sacred syllable, which generates pure knowledge." The sushumna has also been called "Great Path," "Regal Path," "Middle Path," and it has been assimilated to the Tree of Life[9]—life in the eminent sense of immortal life.

It is claimed that after the obstacle has been swept away, the no longer dualistic elementary force that consumes the pingala and the ida finally pours into the sushumna and "lights the fire of death."[10] The texts used the term *death* to describe the traumatic sensation a man experiences at the peak of the magical intercourse with a woman. In both cases it is an experience of transcendence, the breaking through ordinary consciousness, and what ordinary people experience as death. The correspondence between death and initiation (initiation = active death) has always been acknowledged: we can find specific testimonies concerning it in Western antiquity. This correspondence is not allegorical but real: it refers to an ontological change of state within the hierarchy of various states of being. A further correspondence should be acknowledged: when the sushumna is understood as the "Middle Path" (*madhyamarga*), it corresponds to the direction taken by those who, after death, turn toward the unconditioned. All the lateral paths departing from the axis like branches from a tree trunk are believed to lead to other conditioned states of existence.

The abovementioned expansion of consciousness signifies the overcoming of the limitation represented by the waking state, which is conditioned by the physical body. This limitation prevents the perception of the superphysical dimensions of corporeity as well as the occupation of the corresponding seats. Thus Tantric hatha yoga does not merely consist in awakening kundalini. This energy, in fact, becomes a helpful means leading to the realization of the powers hidden in one's body; of the chakras, or occult centers; and of their corresponding forces and principles in the macrocosm. This process, therefore, acquires a transcendent dimension and meaning. Every power in the body becomes known and controlled, in a backward progression in respect to Shakti's cosmic manifestation, until the principle is finally reached.

The following are the general presuppositions of this type of yoga: (1) one must be able to overcome the crisis induced by kundalini's awakening, and not be swept away; (2) one must unite with kundalini; (3) kundalini must be led and guided through the various chakras. This means that a lucid, firm control must be maintained even in the supernatural dimension and in the transphysical states of consciousness. I must emphasize again that if the basic force, or "serpent power," as it has been called, awakens and starts acting randomly, this is still not considered enough. The force must be controlled. Here we find the symbolism of a widow (Shakti in a state of release) who awaits her mate.

There is another important aspect to be considered. When dealing with Tantric cosmology, I referred to a descending phase, *pravritti-marga*, that corresponds to the purely emanative phase of the manifestation, taking place under the aegis of Shakti, who is free of bonds, extroverted, and who finds her limitation at the level of the earth. The next phase, *nirvritti-marga*, involves the "reabsorption" (*laya*) of this Shakti, in terms of a reunion with Shiva. In kundalini yoga, also called *laya yoga*, this process seems to take place *sub specie interioritatis*. Kundalini "awakens" various chakras, but this, per se, is not enough, and we should not consider only the awakening and the attainment of spiritual corporeity. Each of the first six chakras is also seen as the seat of a god and of his shakti. Their awakening is achieved though their sexual union (which clearly corresponds to the gradual removal of the dualistic law of *maya-shakti*). This means that the yogic process involves the transformation of the Shaktic element into Shiva. Likewise, in the ascending phase of the manifestation, or to be precise, at its peak, which corresponds to the seventh chakra, a reference is made to the supreme union of Shiva and Shakti, at a transcendental level. When Tantric Buddhism talks about "allowing various buddhas to enter into the body's chakras" (this is the equivalent of a mating between a god and a goddess in each of these chakras), it obviously agrees with the Tantric Hindu perspective, since a buddha corresponds to the Shaivist luminous element. In Vajrayana the realization of the chakras corresponds to supernatural experiences and to the creation of various limbs of the so-called diamond body (*vajra-rupa*).

Let us proceed now to learn about the various chakras. My main source will be two short treatises, the Shatchakra-Nirupana and the Padukapanchaka, which were translated into English by Arthur Avalon in his book *The Serpent Power*. We find in Avalon's text a clarification of all the elements and symbols attributed by the two treatises to various chakras, and especially to Hindu gods. Unfortunately I must follow the stereotypical and somewhat overly schematic description given by the texts.

The seven chakras are called *muladhara, svadhishthana, manipura, anahata, vishuddha, ajna,* and *sahasrara.* The first five correspond to the "great elements" (tattvas)—earth, water, fire, air, and ether. The sixth chakra, *ajna,* corresponds to the "inner organ" and to the individuating intellectual powers up to and including buddhi. The tattvas that occupy a higher place on the hierarchy correspond to the space between the *ajna-chakra* and *sahasrara-chakra,* which is located at the top of the head. This spot corresponds to the specific and supreme unity and, in mythological accounts, to the peak of Mount Kailasa, the dwelling place of Shiva, who is called "the Lord of the Mountain." As I have said, these centers are located along the spinal cord and its extension. They are portrayed as lotus flowers; each of them has a specific number of petals, which correspond to the "causal letters" (*matrika*) and to the invisible forces of the *natura naturans.* These forces are found united in various ways in the human spiritual corporeity and are manifested as shaping forces and as pranic currents irradiating from each chakra. The number of petals corresponds to the number of these currents. Since, following this way, the connection of the physical body parts is finally achieved, there seems to be an analogy between the chakras and the plexuses found in the human organism. In addition to the letters, a mantra is associated with each chakra, which has a relation with the prevailing power in it. This mantra may be used in the process of awakening. What follows is a summary of the analytical description found in the texts.

MULADHARA-CHAKRA

Corresponding to the sacral-coccygeal plexus, the *muladhara-chakra* is located at the base of the spinal cord (at the tip of the filum terminale), between the anus and the genitals. It has four petals, corresponding to the Sanskrit letters *va, sha, ca,* and *sa.* Its color is yellow. Its mandala is a square, which in turn is the earth's mandala. The earth is the tattva corresponding to this chakra. Its mantra is LAM. This chakra is related to (1) the cohesiveness of physical matter; (2) the *tanmatra* of smell and its corresponding organ; (3) apana, or "down-breath"; and (4) the human skeleton.

This chakra is the seat of the "god of the earth," or of the demiurge (Brahma), and of his Shakti, Dakini. The elephant on

which the mantra LAM is sometimes inscribed represents the bulki-
ness, weight, and stasis characterizing the manifestations of the
earth's tattva. In the middle of the chakra one finds an inverted
triangle, the symbol of the Shakti principle. Inside the triangle one
finds the *svayambhu-linga*, on which the mantra of desire, KLIM, is
written in red. According to a text: "Within it [the triangle] the self-
subsisting reality appears in the form of a linga [phallus]." This
means that the self-subsisting power, in this context, takes the form
of a generating power. Inside the triangle one may also find a
dormant kundalini, wrapped around the linga with three and a half
coils. This serpent obstructs, with its head, "*brahman's* threshold"
and the access to the sushumna, which departs from this chakra's
center.

Various forms of the affective and emotional life of ordinary
people are associated with each chakra. The following are associated with the *muladhara-chakra*: greed (*lobha*), false knowledge, credu-
lity, delusions, and indulgence in coarse and obtuse material
pleasures. The force that induces sleep is also ascribed to this chakra.

SVADHISHTHANA-CHAKRA

Corresponding to the prostatic plexus, the *svadhisthana-chakra* is
located at the base of the genitals. It has six petals, corresponding
to the letters *ba, bha, ma, ya, ra,* and *la.* Its color is white. Its mandala
is a crescent moon, the symbol of the water tattva, which corresponds to this chakra. Its mantra is VAM. This chakra is related to (1)
the contracting force of physical matter; (2) the *tanmatra* of taste and
its corresponding organ; (3) the gripping organs (especially the
hands); (4) the genital and ejaculative functions of the vital force;
and (5) the adipose tissues.

This chakra is the seat of Vishnu, who represents the preserving aspect of the godhead, and of his Shakti, Rakini. The god is
represented as having four arms, holding respectively a shell, a
disk, a lotus, and a mace. The goddess, too, is portrayed with four
arms; her hands hold a trident, a lotus, a drum, and a spear. She has
three eyes, and her countenance is terrifying. The name of this
chakra means (Shakti's) "own-base center." On the other hand, the
mantra VAM is said to be "immaculate and as bright as the moon in
an autumn night." This antithesis refers to the transformation, taking place beyond the earth, of the unleashed power, which is connected to the humid principle (the Hermetic passage from the
"lower-level waters" to the "heavenly waters").

The correspondences on the affective plane are sexual desire, tiredness, aversion, shame, and languor. The force that causes thirst in an ordinary person is ascribed to this chakra.

MANIPURA-CHAKRA

Corresponding to the hypogastric plexus, the *manipura-chakra* is located at the base of the lumbar region, at the level below the navel. It has ten petals, corresponding to the letters *da, dha, na, ta, tha, da, na, pa,* and *pha*.[11] Its color is red. Its mandala is a triangle with swastikas at its angles, which represent the fire tattva, which corresponds to this chakra. Its mantra is RAM. This chakra is related to (1) the expanding force of matter; (2) the *tanmatra* of sight (color and form) and its corresponding organ; (3) the function of defecation; (4) the assimilating and digestive function of the vital force; and (5) the flesh and muscles. *Tejas,* or brilliance, is often associated with this chakra.

Manipura literally means "jeweled city." It is conceived as a "red area of a flame," or as the seat of Rudra (Shiva's equivalent) or as the dissolutive and consuming manifestation of the cosmic power. The god, according to popular iconography, is covered with the ashes collected from the material consumed by the fire; he is portrayed in *vara-mudra* and in *abhaya-mudra,* the double gesture that dispenses favors and dissipates fear.[12] He is portrayed in the company of Lakini, his Shakti, who has three heads and three eyes, and who holds a thunderbolt and a sword in her hands. These images induce us to think that in this chakra the yogic process provokes a combustion. The force of desire, which in the previous chakra existed in a liquid state, is here consumed in a burning, shining substance that is all-pervasive.

The corresponding affective forces are anger (*krodha*), fear, astonishment, violence, and pride. The force that manifests itself in an ordinary person as hunger is associated with this chakra.

ANAHATA-CHAKRA

Corresponding to the cardiac plexus, the *anahata-chakra* is located at the level of the heart. It has twelve petals, corresponding to the letters *ka, kha, ga, gha, na, ca, cha, ja, jha, jna, ta,* and *tha.* Its color is dark gray. According to a Vedantic interpretation, gray is the color of smoke engulfing a living being's atman (*jivatma*) prior to his enlightenment. The Upanishads claim that the atman is located in the deepest recesses of the heart, which is believed to be the seat of the divine as well as the center of one's personality. Its mandala is a six-point star, formed by two inverted triangles in perfect equilibrium. This is also the symbol of the air tattva, which corresponds to this chakra. Its mantra is YAM. This chakra is related to (1) movement in physical reality; (2) the *tanmatra* of touch and its corresponding organ (skin); (3) the male sexual organ; (4) the swallowing and digestive functions of the vital force; and (5) the blood system.

This is the seat of the god Isha, the "Lord," who is the manifestation of the primordial power in the form of a personal god (this manifestation is reflected in the *atma* as the principle of the individual's personality). This god, too, is portrayed in the double gesture of driving away fear and of granting favors, and so is Kakini, his Shakti, "filled with the sweet nectar of immortality." The name of this chakra derives from the fact that in it, the yogins are able to perceive the "unstruck sound," which is associated with "the life stream in the jiva." The texts offer some further images. Inside the hexagonal star, there is, just as in the *muladhara-chakra*, an inverted triangle, representing the goddess's yoni (sexual organ). This triangle too contains Shiva's phallus, which is a golden *vanalinga*. On the linga we find inscribed the symbol of the moon, which is dominated by the *bindu*, the one and simple dot. Under the linga we find an image of the vital principle *(hamsah)*, which in this context assumes the meaning of the superpersonal I, aptly described in the Bhagavad-Gita as "a still flame in a windless place." In this description, it is clear that the general views contained in the Upanishads about the heart as the center of the human being and as the seat of the *atma* mingle with specifically Tantric views.

The correspondences on the affective plane are hope, anxiety, apprehension, doubt, remorse, and hesitation. The mantra YAM is inscribed on a black antelope, which symbolizes the immaterial speed of the wind.

VISHUDDHA-CHAKRA

Corresponding to the larynx, the *vishuddha-chakra* is located on the axis of the spinal cord, at the level of the throat, in the place in which the spinal cord becomes the medulla oblongata. It has sixteen petals, which correspond to sixteen letters of the Sanskrit alphabet. Its color is bright, shining white. Its mandala is a circle, which symbolizes ether, to which it corresponds. Its mantra is HAM. It is related to (1) the expanding force of physical reality; (2) the *tanmatra* of sound and the sense of hearing; (3) the expression of vital energy; (4) the mouth; and (5) the skin.

In this center, the androgynous god Sadashiva's body is portrayed half white as snow (in other descriptions it is of a silver color) and half golden. He is carried by an animal that is half lion and half bull. The -shiva suffix of this god's name alludes to the "eternal being," and therefore to an extrasamsaric condition. Next to this god is his Shakti, Sakini, who is white and cold. It is said that her form is that of a "light unto herself."[13] This signifies that, at this level, Shiva's quality has been transfused into Shakti. The region of this chakra is described as a lunar and ethereal region (the ethereal light that turns the night into day) and as the threshold of the "Great Liberation." It has been said that while dwelling in it, *atma* sees itself in everything and dominates the three dimensions of time (past, present, and future). The mantra HAM, in this chakra's representations, is carried by a white elephant. This may represent the transformation of what in the *muladhara-chakra* characterizes the earth tattva, namely, ether (*akasha*), understood in terms of spatial consciousness, as opposed to material nontransparent density.

The correspondences on the affective plane are affection, sadness, respect, devotion, happiness, regret, and relationships.

AJNA-CHAKRA

Corresponding to the cavernous plexus, the *ajna-chakra* is located in the middle of the head, at the level of the eyebrows. It has two petals, which correspond to the letters *ha* and *ksha*. Its color is a dazzling white blaze. Its mantra is AUM. It is related to (1) the cerebellum; (2) the marrow; (3) "the inner organ," which includes buddhi, manas, and ahamkara; and (4) *sukshma-prakriti,* which on a macrocosmic level is the root of all the powers of nature considered in its subtle dimension.

Inside this chakra's inverted triangle the goddess Hakini, who looks like Kali, is represented. She is Shiva's bride at the level of his highest manifestation (Paramshiva). Hakini's complexion is white, and she appears intoxicated by the "ambrosia," or nectar of immortality. She has six faces and six arms. Two of her hands are repeating the mudras that exorcise fears and dispense favors, while the other hands are holding symbolic objects: a rosary, a skull, a small drum, and a book. *Ajna-chakra* literally means "command wheel." It is located in the same place as the *urna,* the frontal stone that in Hindu iconography alludes to the third eye, or to Shiva's eye. This eye acts as a thunderbolt (*vajra*). The texts attribute to it a cyclical or "cyclopic" transcendent vision. An analogous meaning is conveyed in the representation of an inverted triangle that contains a linga in the shape of a thunderbolt or of a diamond; this triangle symbolizes the goddess and the yoni, the female sexual organ. Shiva's virility penetrates Shakti in the form of *vajra*, the thunderbolt force, and it manifests itself in every magical command. Its counterpart is the portrayal of the "inner spirit" (*antaratma*), which shines like a flame right above the linga (in this context called *itara-linga*); in its light "everything that is included in the manifestation"[14] becomes clearly visible. There is more to this symbolism. Above the inverted triangle we find the moon surmounted by the *bindu*. In the *bindu*, according to a commentary, there is "an infinite space, shining with the splendor of countless suns."[15] This region is the dwelling place of the "Lord who is beyond peacefulness" (this alludes to a state higher than the mere "ether of consciousness"), whose body is made of lightning. This is the threshold of the pure tattvas.

MANAS-CHAKRA AND SOMA-CHAKRA

The Tantric texts mention two minor centers located in the proximity of the *ajna-chakra*. The first is called *manas-chakra* and has six petals. As the name implies, it is related to the mental aspect of the jiva; to the formation and representation of ideas, which are connected to the afferent sensory system; and to the imaginative faculty, which is manifested even in dreams and in hallucinations. As far as this chakra's awakening is concerned, if the yogic process has not unfolded properly, there is the danger of incurring hallucinations and of experiencing a chaotic clairvoyance.

The second minor center is called *soma-chakra*. It has sixteen petals and is located in the middle of the brain, above the minor center I have just described. The descriptions of its functions are not very accurate. This center is believed to relate to some forms of creative idealizations and to anything related to a thought process unfolding in a rigorously logical fashion. Self-control is associated with this chakra, as are various feelings and dispositions of the jiva's ordinary life, such as compassion, generosity, renunciation, determination, and seriousness.

THE SEVEN FORMS OF THE CAUSAL BODY

In the middle of the forehead there is a twelve-petaled white lotus, which is associated with the pure tattvas. According to popular symbolism, this is not really a true chakra, but rather a region that

155

includes (1) the Great Goddess's inverted triangle, which is here called *a-ka-tha*. These are three Sanskrit letters corresponding to the three sides of the triangle. They symbolize the elements of the triad included in the *parabindu*, which is the transcendental unity (sun, moon, fire, and other related triads are also employed); (2) a space made of sound, in which the *parabindu* becomes the primordial motion, believed to be a sound; (3) "the area surrounding the altar" (the "Eternal Master," who is gigantic, imposing, and "looking like a silver mountain,"[16] sits on this altar "of the color of bright red gems"); and (4) *hamsah* in its supreme and "eternal" expression. The latter is the equivalent of the union between Shiva (*ham*) and Shakti *(sah)*, which constitutes the first tattva on the transcendent hierarchy.

This region is called "residence without foundations" and indicates the self-subsisting power that characterizes the pure tattvas. The texts suggest that here the yogins realize the seven forms of the causal body, which correspond to the seven stages of pure power (Shiva-Shakti, *nada, bindu, tribindu,* sattva, rajas, tamas). If such a body receives the name of *karanavantara-karira* (intermediate and successive causal body), this must be understood in relation to the immobile cause of which it represents the primordial manifestation, made of pure act. In this region, too, we find the double mudra of dissipating fear and granting favors.

SAHASRARA-CHAKRA

Located on the head, above the fontanel, the *sahasrara-chakra* is called the "thousand-petaled lotus," but this number does not correspond to the actual pranic currents, as was the case in the other chakras; this number, rather, signifies greatness. According to some, since the number one thousand equals fifty multiplied by twenty, it symbolizes the multiplication or further power of the fifty letters of the Sanskrit alphabet. It is also believed that these letters, variously distributed in the six lower chakras, are gathered in the *sahasrara-chakra*. In this chakra we find again the symbol of the great Shakti's inverted triangle. Its counterpart this time is no longer a linga but rather the "supreme dot" (*parabindu*), understood in the terms of emptiness (*shunya*). Emptiness symbolizes the unconditioned and the immaterial simplicity of a pure transcendent enlightenment, in which the limitations of every conditioned state have been removed. "Fullness," on the contrary, signifies the whole of the tattvas in their immanent aspect, which is connected to the manifestation and variously articulated. In the *sahasrara-chakra*, Shakti finally becomes, without any residual, *chidrupini*. She takes the form of Shiva, and therefore becomes resolved and freed. She becomes one with her "bridegroom's body," to form a union higher than either one. This union corresponds to Vajrayana's *mahasukha-kaya*, which is the state beyond the unilaterally conceived transcendent nirvana.

The *sahasrara-chakra* is called a chakra only for practical purposes. In reality it is not a "center" like the others. It is situated outside the body, in the spot where the axial line goes beyond the cranium. Since the body corresponds to the universe, the *sahasrara-chakra*, or the dimension of transcendence that is beyond the universe, is analogically located above the head.

The description of the chakras given in the Tantras is multifaceted. First of all, what has been considered is the correspondence of the chakras with various plexuses, functions, and forces of the human organism. This means that in these plexuses, functions, and forces, there are dormant forms of consciousness, which are associated with various gods presiding over bodily activities. Second, the first five chakras are believed to correspond to as many elements (tattvas). This correspondence may constitute a foundation for the knowledge or the experience of them, simply by focusing dhyana or *samyama* on any given chakra.

Most likely, the mantras associated with each chakra are given to the apprentice for practical purposes: the awakening of the chakras may be facilitated by the use of the mantra that apppears in its visualization.

As far as the various divinities associated with each chakra are concerned, it may well be said that the contemplation of them and of their attributes may prepare the way for the awakening. This is obviously contingent on the quality of the contemplation to be found in the worshiper of a particular deity. The opposite process may also take place: if a god that was realized in dhyana is instrumental in a chakra's awakening, this awakening, in turn, may be helpful to "demythologize" this god and to enable the apprentice to see his essence as a corresponding formless state, which is proper to initiatory knowledge.

The seven chakras reproduce the Septenary, or the Ebdomades, spoken of in several Mysteriosophic and initiatory traditions. These traditions mention a planetary hierarchy; heavenly journeys; the ascent through seven spheres; seven levels, or degrees, of initiation (e.g., Mithra's mysteries); and alchemical transformations of "prime matter,"[17] associated with the planets. All of these things symbolize experiences analogous to the ones found in hatha yoga (ascent through the chakras). As I have said before, these experiences should not be "psychologized," but rather should be understood in terms of a cosmic expansion of consciousness. In the course of the ascent along sushumna, one takes on the bodies of various gods and claims possession of seats (*lokas*) beyond the phenomenal world, called *bhur-loka, bhuvar-loka, svar-loka, jana-loka, tapar-loka,* and *mahar-loka.*

Generally speaking, a particular type of knowledge typical of the corresponding tattva is attributed to each awakened chakra. For instance, the spheres or worlds of fire, water, air, and ether, which are the first tattvas beyond the earth, are considered to be transformations of the experiences of nature and also to be living beings, which have a correspondence with the tattva manifested in it. Thus, the lower chakras are supposed to provide knowledge of the laws and of the forces acting in the elementary aspects of nature. The chakra located at the solar plexus confers the knowledge of the character and of the dispositions of human beings. The chakras at the heart and at the larynx allow the apprentice to detect the feelings and thoughts of other people. This obviously presupposes the acquired capability of relocating one's consciousness to various areas of the subtle body. From a magical point of view, the power over an element that a person may acquire is also supposed to confer dominion over the manifestations of that element in the external world, because of the substantial and ontological unity of the principles involved.

It would be interesting to look for the correspondence between the Tantric view of kundalini and the teachings and symbols of other traditions, but this would take us too far off. I will only suggest here that the *ureus,* the serpent that in Egyptian art is worn by the king as a diadem, probably symbolizes the same life force.[18] Also, when the Hermetists spoke of the "philosopher's basilisk," which as a thunderbolt burns every "imperfect metal," or of the "Dry Way," we may probably see in these symbols a reference to kundalini's awakening. Other correspondences could be found concerning the basic center or *muladhara-chakra*[19] in both the East and the West.

· XI ·

TECHNIQUES EMPLOYED TO AWAKEN THE SERPENT POWER

Yoga's sadhana is mainly based on breath and on breath control (pranayama). Pranayama is far from being a prerogative of Tantrism alone. It is also found in classical yoga. Patañjali describes it as "the cutting off of the flow of inhalation and exhalation after assuming a steady and comfortable position."[1] A real suspension of breath (*viccheda*) takes place only in the last stages of the yogic practice, which even in subsequent stages is referred to as pranayama. In any event, breath control and its suspension can be used for very different purposes.[2] Tantric yoga employs pranayama in order to awaken kundalini, while dhyana yoga uses it to regulate and to suspend the flow of mental activities.

This does not prevent hatha yoga from employing breath suspension in preliminary practices. Thus pranayama may be associated with procedures through which one attempts to elevate consciousness to the seats that correspond to the body's deepest levels of corporeity. The premise here consists in a relationship between various breathing rhythms and those seats. The most immediate factor is breath according to a rhythm proper to waking consciousness, which is essentially connected to mental activities. In this form, breathing has two characteristics. First, it is as arrhythmic and unmethodical as the mental and the emotional life of ordinary people. Second, there is a disproportion between the inspiratory and the expiratory phases, since their duration usually varies.

The starting point of these practices consists in the "undertaking of prana's seat," which is also referred to as "riding the *hamsah* bird." The word *hamsah* refers to the vital principle in its particular relationship with breath and with prana (the two syllables of the word refer to inhaling and exhaling, respectively). The representation of *hamsah* as a bird alludes to the volatile and unstable rhythm of ordinary breathing, which comes in and goes out countless times, day and night, and to the flighty and elusive nature of the vital principle present in humankind. It is said that yoga's power is capable of transforming *hamsah*'s nature and of overcoming its birdlike mobility by rendering it non-terrestrial.

I have previously explained that prana is not ordinary breathing, but breathing considered in its subtle and living dimension. This essential point is often forgotten in the Western popularization of yoga, in which pranayama is often misrepresented as a sort of breathing exercise (that yoga may prove beneficial in ordinary life even in this form does not invalidate my contention). The texts describe the dematerialization, internalization, and essential function of breath that lead to an experience of prana. The texts' reference to a specific prana aimed at various parts of the body clearly indicates that they do not employ the term in its ordinary sense.

Thus the expression "riding the *hamsah* bird" refers to the transformation of ordinary breath into living breath. The first step of the pranayama process consists in assuming a different breathing rhythm, which is increasingly calm, even, deep, and slow, as well as different from the rhythm characterizing the waking state. This technique is used to break down the blocked doors of the subconscious. The texts suggest the choice, first and foremost, of the rhythm $2t$–t–$2t$, which comprises an inhalation (*puraka*) lasting, for example, six seconds; a retention of breath (*kumbhaka*) lasting half that time (e.g., for three seconds); and finally, an expiration (*rechaka*) lasting six seconds, followed by a three-second abstention from breath, and so on. Time may be measured by the count of one's heartbeats or by the mental recitation of a mantra. Little by little, the rhythm becomes slower, effortless, simply through a mental action. Every single phase or degree in this progression should be sufficiently consolidated, so that the apprentice may be able to achieve it at will, and to adopt it as natural rhythm, only a few minutes into the practice. In this way, the apprentice does not need to avert his attention from the direction and the control of what constitutes pranayama's physical aspect.

When the exercise is performed in the proper way, it facilitates the shift of the apprentice's consciousness seat. This shift is referred to as "to reenter" or "to move into an inner state." Without exaggerations, it is said that making the inspiration and expiration even through the $2t$–t–$2t$ rhythm allows one to drink from the source of immortality, which is located in the "sun." In any event, the effect of the first change of state brought about by pranayama consists in feeling a calm and solar presence in one's life. We can now begin to understand why this transformation, or descent, is also said to be a reentering. In the seat that in the common person is that of dissipation in sleep and in torpor, the values are inverted. The seat reveals itself to be that of "being within oneself," in a state of perfect calm and lucidity, compared to which waking consciousness is a "being outside oneself," in a world of distractions and of restlessness.

More specifically, moving into the heart's seat either implies or occasions (the difference depends on the methods employed)[3] the suspension (or the "slaying") of manas, which is the organ responsible for discursive thought, the creation of ideas, and mental associations, which are all "psychological" functions. "To slay manas in one's heart" is a recurrent theme in the Upanishads. In the Maitri-Upanishad we read: "So long the mind [manas] should be confined, till in the heart it meets its end. That is both knowledge and release! All else is but a string of words!"[4] And also: "Holding his body steady with the three upper parts erect, and causing the senses with the mind to enter into the heart, a wise man with the Brahma-boat should cross over all the fear-bringing streams [of samsara]."[5] The psychological states are the following: What first takes place is the occurrence of clear thoughts interconnected by activities produced by the I, which intervenes and arranges them in different patterns. Second, we have the arising of the spontaneous and unintentional associations of ideas, which takes place in a state of semiconsciousness. Third, we have a cessation of mentally "spoken" thoughts and a decrease in mental images, which become progressively sporadic and rare. Following these stages, an ordinary person's manas is consumed in sleep. A yogin's manas, instead, is replaced with states leading to superconsciousness, which is proper to the heart's chakra.

Further stages of pranayama involve an increasingly slower rhythm of breathing, until breath ceases. There is an area in which all of this is supposed to take place. In this area, which extends beyond the cardiac region in the direction of the *muladhara-chakra*, some further changes of state are believed to occur. If one is able to organically become part of this development and to carry it further, he would eventually come across the state that corresponds, on the physical plane, to the skeleton. In this state (the "earth" of the human body), breathing stops and consciousness appears as scorching and abyssal heat. Some texts talk about the apparition of a skeleton, "as wide as the universe," consisting of a white thunderbolt. The terminal point is self-centeredness, or a sense of an absolute "I AM," or "I," which is the residue of *hamsah* or of prana, which has now become a self-consuming force. Upon the overcoming of this limitation, kundalini awakens and enters into the sushumna.[6]

This process will unfold naturally, through a series of various degrees, after the seat of prana has been occupied, and after the *hamsah* bird has been firmly restrained. The intensity of concentration on a specific central, detached spot, made of light, could facilitate the passage from one phase to the other. At a certain moment the change in the breath's rhythm and its suspension would turn from cause into effect, almost in the sense of a physical reflex of an absolute stillness and unity, which are realized inwardly.[7] This is one aspect of the process. Another aspect corresponds to the Taoist symbol of a dragon that takes to flight into ether, as well as to Mithras, who grabs the bull by the horns and begins to ride on it. The animal begins to run widely, but Mithras does not let go his grip, and when the bull, exhausted, comes to a halt, he slays it.[8] This last phase could correspond to the aforesaid breaking point, and also to the symbol of Phineus's spear-thrust, which I have associated with the initiatory Tantric sexual practices. If the process, in this second aspect, is interpreted in terms of pranayama, it is believed to consist in the slowing down of normal breathing, which is spontaneous, without any spiritual intervention, while the apprentice remains self-aware during the subtle intensification of power. If left "unchanged," breathing would change rhythm by itself, as in the case of people who become numb or fall asleep. The terms *flight* and *race* refer to the experience of the ensuing change of states, if consciousness persists.

In both aspects of practice, we should consider two essential issues: (1) a total inner stillness, or a subtle self-awareness, which does not disturb the natural development and transformation of the breathing states, and (2) the capability to overcome organic fear.

Exercises of this kind should be initiated and carried out with an adequate state of mind. In the twofold path, which I have characterized as normal, or as natural, the primary factor is one's inner orientation. If sadhana is not practiced with an open, wide, unlimited, and bright mind, free from worldly concerns, it will be difficult to cross the threshold of consciousness and to adapt to the first change of state. This state of mind can be propitiated or strengthened through suitable images that evoke the majesty, superior calmness, and cosmic dimension of nature as well as the impersonal and boundless elements contained in it.

In kundalini yoga the twofold "natural" procedure is not the only one adopted. Active interventions, which are a particular expression of both the vital breath and of the magical imagination, are contemplated at higher levels, as one strives to remain in a state of centrality and of a calm and solar presence in this earthly life. These higher levels presuppose a healthy and strong physical organism and a heart in good condition. Second, it is necessary to train in order to optimize physical breathing and to fully exploit the lungs' capacity. The lower part of the lungs should be filled by lowering the diaphragm and by expanding the frontal part of the abdomen; then the middle part of the lungs should be filled by elevating the sternum and by stretching the lower ribs. Finally, the higher part of the lungs should be filled by pushing the chest out and by pulling the shoulders back. One should then breath not through the mouth but through the nose. These three phases eventually must be unified in one continuous and spontaneous motion.

I have already mentioned that Patañjali puts the realization of asana before pranayama. One of the most popular asanas in Hindu yoga is *siddha-asana,* as the reader may well recall. The yogin sits with the neck and torso upright, cross-legged. The left heel touches the perineum, which is the area where the *muladhara-chakra* is located and where the spinal cord ends (according to some texts it should obstruct the anal orifice). The right heel leans on the folded left leg, possibly touching the genitals and covering the penis's orifice. The hands are held horizontally, palms facing upward, the right hand under the left one, below the solar plexus. Such a posture should guarantee a high degree of stability. Another frequently used asana differs from *siddha-asana* only in that the hands rest on the knees; the fingers are stretched with the exception of thumb and of the index, forming an O. In ancient Western traditions, bodily postures similar to Hindu asanas can also be found. A position having the dignity of an asana that is found in Egyptian iconography consisted in sitting upright on a throne, holding the legs together, and keeping the arms at a right angle, as they lean on the throne's armrests.

As far as the esoteric dimension of the asanas is concerned, I have already mentioned that a preliminary contemplation, leading the apprentice to identify with a deity, is required. This contemplation introduces the apprentice to the esoteric meaning of each asana. Bodily postures should be experienced as symbols and as divine seals. When one assumes a given position, he should do it with the intention of becoming the living statue of a god.

When the members of the body are arranged in an asana, a distinct fluid state (which can also be defined as a fluid sense of well-being) can be perceived, even if the apprentice has not developed the subtle sensibility to a high degree. This state determines the stopping of the circulation of the body's pranic currents. Another relevant factor is the evocation and the ensuing "freezing" of the "fluid state of immobility." The neutrality and the lucid fixedness of a mind that is free from mental formations should be infused into the body through a magical image, such as the "statue of a god." This process is important from a material point of view as well, since it allows the apprentice to maintain a still bodily posture for a long time without ever getting tired or sore (especially in the spinal cord), in virtue of an occult command transmitted to the physical organism.

What I have said so far concerns the preliminary realization of an asana. Next, I will discuss specific practices of kundalini yoga. There are two levels in these practices: (1) the pranic saturation of the body and (2) the awakening of the serpent power.

PRANIC SATURATION OF THE BODY

It is said that the first thing to do is to saturate the body with prana, just as electricity saturates a condenser. Needless to say, prana has nothing to do with oxygen. The apprentice is supposed to absorb prana, and not the oxygen found in the air. This process can be separated from the physical breathing function, since the absorption of prana can take place without breathing, or better, during the exhalation phase. Therefore, the process takes place on the plane of invisible corporeity and of its energies. The apprentice is told to accumulate, by inhaling, the fire power or radiant energy (*tejas*).

1. Respiration according to the $2t$–t–$2t$ rhythm must be animated by the perception of breath as a current of bright light, coming

and going. This current must be visualized in the event one does not have a direct experience of this breath. Eventually, the current of light becomes more intense and more saturated, and it feeds the chakra located at the region of the heart, which corresponds to the Shaivist I, just like a flame that grows taller after being blown on by the bellows.

2. Another exercise that attempts to achieve the same results consists in the already-mentioned identification of one's body with a particular deity: "Visualize the physical body as being internally vacuous, like the inside of an empty sheath, transparent and uncloudedly radiant." Following the breathing pace, the visualized figure is expanded to the size of a mountain, and then, during exhalation, reduced to the size of a small seed.[9]

3. A third exercise consists in imagining rays of light radiating from the pores of one's body during exhalation and in their reentering the body and filling the physical organism during inhalation. This exercise is complicated by the projection and ensuing reabsorption of sacred syllables, which are eventually changed into wrathful deities.[10]

The systematic repetition of the exercises causes the physical rhythm of breathing to turn into the mere vehicle of a mental rhythm, which eventually becomes predominant and autonomous. This is achieved either through a pranic respiration, which is performed not only with the throat but with the whole body; or through retention of breath; or through the inner inversion of the normal phases of breathing.[11] Especially in Taoism, this is a slow, deep, silent respiration, "resembling that of an embryo," and it is performed with the entire body, starting from the soles of the feet. The consequence of this exercise is the valorization of the vital energy (the Taoist equivalent of prana is *chi*, or "ethereal fluid"); its rhythm also becomes substantially immaterial.

4. The technique of reversal of breath is mentioned in the Bhagavad-Gita (4:29) in the following terms: "Some offer their out-flowing breath into the breath that flows in; and the in-flowing breath into the breath that flows out." Physical breathing here has two inverted meanings. Inhaling should be experienced as a letting go and as becoming dissolved; exhaling should be experienced as a rising and a summoning of strengths. An intimate sense of continuity ought to unite the two phases. It is important to induce a growing imbalance and an excess of the second phase.

One should therefore let oneself go when inhaling, in order to arise more decisively with each exhalation. The purpose of this exercise is to turn the body into an oversaturated condenser of pranic energy.

5. The goal of "breathing with a progressive rhythm" is not dissimilar from this purpose. It consists in breathing from alternate nostrils according to the following rhythm: inhale = t; retention = $4t$; exhale = $2t$. This is done while reciting a mantra.

For instance: the right nostril is blocked (at first by pressing it with a finger, and eventually with an inner command) and one inhales from the left nostril for the duration of the repetition of a mantra for eight times, all the while feeling the current flowing in the ida. Breath is then retained for the time necessary to repeat the same mantra thirty-two times. Then the left nostril is blocked and one exhales with the right nostril through the pingala for sixteen repetitions of the mantra. This respiration is repeated numerous times. After that, one reverses the order by inhaling with the right nostril and by exhaling with the left the same number of times. Third, one breathes with that rhythm and with both nostrils the same number of times.

The indicated times to repeat this exercise are dawn, noon, evening, and midnight. The long period of retention of breath, which characterizes this practice, promotes the process of transformation of energies, the fusion of prana and apana, and the production of magic heat. These things take place as the rhythm becomes increasingly slow, deep, and silent. A word of caution is issued: "Breath needs to be tamed gradually, as one does a wild beast, otherwise it will kill the apprentice." At first, a person who practices pranayama might experience chills in the body and a sense of swooning. As practice is integrated with the perfect realization of its subtle dimension and of its inner meaning, what is considered a natural state in a superior order is produced. The texts, for instance, say that kumbhaka [12] is not a state that is achieved only with extreme effort or with hard self-discipline, but that it is rather "the normal state of the spirit." It is breathing that appears to be abnormal. It is also said that kumbhaka increases the stability and strength of the apprentice.

On a physical plane, the effects of these exercises are the opposite of the effects produced by any discipline that promotes mortification of the body:

The signs of hatha yoga's perfection are the following: the body becomes smooth, and the speech eloquent. One can hear inner sounds; the eyes become clear and shining; the organism becomes free from any ailments; semen is concentrated; the digestive fire and the various currents of breath are purified.[13]

In a Tantric Tibetan text the inner states accompanying the first practices of pranic supersaturation of the organism are described in these terms:

Something akin to heat is produced at first; second, blissfulness is experienced; third, the mind assumes its natural state. Then the forming of thoughts ceases automatically, and phenomena, appearing like smoke, mirages, and fireflies, along with something resembling a cloudless sky, are seen.[14]

THE AWAKENING OF THE SERPENT POWER

After a certain time has been devoted to the exercises leading to the pranic supersaturation of the body, the apprentice enters the phase in which the exercises aimed at kundalini's awakening are practiced. One should first find some sort of hermitage, a deserted place, as far as possible from cities and villages. A mountain or even an island is considered the most favorable place.[15] During the most intensive period of the cycle, the apprentice should avoid seeing anyone. Isolation is considered an optimal condition in the preliminary phases as well; it is believed to sharpen the senses and spiritual discernment and to foster inner peace. One should not share with anybody, with the exception of one's guru, what he is doing and what he is planning to do, much less the results or the effects of practice. "The gods love secrecy," and, "A yogi who is desirous of developing siddhis should keep this hatha yoga strictly secret, for only then will he have success. All his efforts will be in vain if he reveals everything without discrimination."[16] It is also important to avoid unnecessary exertions and to adopt a healthy diet. Vegetarianism is strongly encouraged; although in Tibet it is scarcely practiced, it is mandatory for Hindu yogins. For obvious reasons, sexual abstinence as well ought to be practiced, considering that this practice requires the possession and transformation of that power of which the sexual energy is the material manifestation. It is necessary to achieve a state of both physical and fluid calm. In the ritual position advocated by the texts the apprentice should sit facing north.

The care of the apprentice to become isolated from the world, and to create around himself a wall of physical and mental silence, should be accompanied by the contact with those spiritual influences that are related to the tradition of teaching. The following is a propitiatory mental ritual that precedes every exercise. The apprentice imagines his own teacher to sit above his head in his same asana. Above his teacher, still in the same position, one should imagine the preceding representative in the initiatory chain, and so on. All of these teachers form a vertical line of similar figures, one on top of the other, reaching to heaven. This line gradually turns into light and eventually becomes confused with the "original teacher," who symbolizes the nonhuman spiritual influence that radiates along the chain.

In the operative phase one habitually proceeds to empty his body. The body must be thought to be an empty shell, almost as if it were made of a luminous, transparent membrane of an immaterial thinness. The power of the visualizing concentration should be such that, forgetful of his own body, the apprentice should only see this image and identify with it. Within this empty shell one should visualize the three main arteries: the pingala, ida, and sushumna.

The symbol of a motionless Shiva holding a scepter and surrounded by Shakti as if by a fiery dress corresponds to both the pranic supersaturation of the body and to the central power that animates it and that projects the proper figures, symbols, and mantras. The Shaktic dimension of this element is sometimes emphasized through a procedure analogous to the one in which the apprentice spends long periods of time with a woman whom he may desire and yet not possess. One of these exercises consists in visualizing before oneself the "occult bride," Shakti, as a real female figure, endowed with several beautiful traits that are capable of arousing a strong passionate desire in her beholders. The figure is then gradually absorbed into the apprentice.

Hatha yoga distinguishes the simple retention of breath from the "great retention" (mahakevala-kumbhaka). The former is the retention of breath occurring between inspiration and expiration; the latter is a prolonged and uninterrupted one. The former is related to the equalizing breathing pattern 2t–t–2t, or to the progressive breathing t–4t–2t. Inspiration through the pingala and expiration through the ida, and vice versa, may also be applied to the simple rhythm 2t–t–2t. A text outlines the proper technique for the simple retention: inspiration through the ida (left nostril), followed by retention of breath, expiration through the pingala and actualization of *kumbhaka*, which is the prolonged retention. This exercise should be repeated four times a day (early in the morning, noon, evening, and midnight), starting with ten *kumbhakas* per exercise, and building up to eighty *kumbhakas*, by increases of fives. Thus every day one will perform 320 *kumbhakas* in all. The body's perspiration and light trembling indicate the limit that may be reached during breath retention, with the help of an obedient and well-disposed organism. As far as the great retention is concerned, it can be associated with the physical closing of all the body's orifices. The lower orifices (anal and genital) are blocked by the heels if *siddha-asana* is perfectly performed. The other orifices can be closed with the hands: the ears with the thumbs, the eyes with the index and middle fingers, the nostrils with the ring fingers, the two sides of the mouth with the little fingers (this is the so-called *shanmukkhi-mudra*). Later on, this closing can be obtained as a natural consequence of the inner states that have been achieved; only then will the closing maximize its efficacy.

From simple retention one proceeds, through several degrees, to the great retention. In the Hindu Tantric texts it is associated with the use of the mantras HAMSAH and HUM, which are related, respectively, to prana and apana. By inhaling deeply and by animating the pranic current with HAMSAH, the apprentice imagines the current rushing toward the *muladhara-chakra*. According to some texts, the physiological counterpart is a progressive contraction of the anal orifice, followed by a contraction in the torso-cardiac region, when inspiration stops. The contraction of the sphincter is extended to the filum terminale, which is located around the *muladhara-chakra*.[17] When inspiration ends and the phase of breath retention begins, concentration on prana must be intensified according to the various phases of the preliminary exercises: the luminous phase, the warmth phase (corresponding to deep sleep), and the phase that is beyond everything else. The apprentice should go from the mantra HAMSAH to the mantra HUM, which is kundalini's mantra as well. All this is repeated a few times. This exercise is resumed during the day, but it is practiced with less frequency once the rhythm becomes slower and the retention of breath becomes longer, since in this period various transformations, as well as the magical warmth that will awaken kundalini, are produced. Even if one is not busy performing any actions, during the day the mind should be gathered and any eventual partial achievements should be consolidated. During this period sleep becomes like a short nap, even if one sleeps for hours.

In the great retention the abovementioned process is strengthened. Prana produces a kind of vortex, which spins faster and faster until a short circuit occurs, which determines the removal of what blocks *"brahman's* threshold" as well as the awakened serpent power's entrance into the sushumna.[18]

The characteristic physical phenomenon (besides the already-mentioned symptoms such as perspiration and shivers) is a particular sense of lightness, which is not just a mere subjective impression, since in these states one is able to levitate.[19] In order to understand a supernatural phenomenon such as levitation, it should be remembered that a body's weight is subject to the law of gravity. This law, in turn, depends on a broader law, which encompasses not only the physical bodies' attraction but their mutual repelling as well. Attraction (which is manifested in weight), may generate repulsion (which is manifested in levitation) by virtue of a change of polarity determined by pranayama, since this involves an inversion of pranic currents.[20]

From a subjective point of view, the awakening is preannounced by certain sounds, which have been compared to the intense buzz of a swarm of bees, and to the cracking of thunder. It may also be noticed that the mantra employed (HUM) is similar to the sound that was produced at the peak of Mithraic initiations. In relation to the great retention, this image is given: One should begin to sink into retained breath as if a circle was closing in. Then, gathering up one's strength, overcoming all fears, by realizing "I am Her," one should jump. If the jump was sufficient and if "the mind took the form of that knowledge," ("I am Her") one will find himself outside the circle, safe and well. The syncope of breath will generate the principle of a new life, made of *amrita*, which permeates the body. This is the regeneration produced by the Shaivist principle of *svayambhu-linga*, which is stronger than death. From the point of view of ordinary people, the yogin, through the *kuvala-kumbhaka*, faces a deadly trial; he could virtually kill himself, since this process leads to asphyxiation.[21] Thus the yogin becomes superior to life itself, since he continues to exist through a residue of energy that survives the point in which kundalini, having entered the sushumna, "lights the fire of death."[22]

The most important stage reached by the serpent power is that of an immediate and absolute identification: SA'M ("I am Her"). If one is not up to it, everything will be in vain. As we shall see in

Appendix Two, this is almost the same trial that awaits those who try to achieve the Great Liberation in the afterlife. It has been said that the only person qualified to practice kundalini yoga is a *shuddhabuddhisvabhana*, one whose substance consists in the pure principle of intellectual determination (buddhi) in its proper form. This form is the aspect in which buddhi is on the borderline between the individual and superindividual dimensions, and is free from prakriti. This is another way to refer to Shiva's virility and to the semen produced by the *svayambhu-linga*. This form can be associated with the braveness and boldness that are the fundamental prerequisites not only for the experiences of viras but for yoga in general.[23]

Some texts of Tibetan Tantrism mention technical details pertaining to special visualizations. I will mention two exercises. The starting point in both exercises is the realization of the form of the vacuous body, which contains the caduceus formed by the pingala, ida, and sushumna.

In the course of the first exercise, some letters of the Tibetan alphabet are used as the support and as the instruments of the magical imagination. These letters are the short *a*, which corresponds to Shakti, and the long *a*, written *ham* and pronounced *hum*, which corresponds to Shiva. The reader should be aware that these are letters of the Tibetan and not of the Sanskrit alphabet; therefore, one should not mistake *hum* for the Sanskrit word that characterizes kundalini's mantra. On the contrary, *hum* (written *ham*) corresponds to the personal pronoun *I* and to the male Shaivist principle. The two letters, shown in the illustration above, must be visualized in this fashion. The feminine *a* is inside the *muladhara-chakra*, at the base of the spine, and is brown. The masculine *a* is located in the *sahasrara-chakra*, at the top of the head, and is white. In the course of the exercise, one performs a short retention of breath between inspiration and expiration. During inspiration the apprentice should visualize his breath to run down, through the pingala and ida, and finally to reach the letter *a* that is located in the *muladhara-chakra*. When the breath reaches the *muladhara-chakra*, the letter takes on a more vivid color and becomes bright red, just like a fiery charcoal turning into flame. The apprentice is supposed to concentrate on this image and to feed it with prana especially during the retention of breath. After that, he must exhale, while imagining his breath ascending along the sushumna in the form of a bluish current.

In a second set of exercises the apprentice must imagine a vivid, vertical flame rising vortically from the letter *a* located in the basal center (chakra). After each breath this flame grows by an inch, so that after ten complete breaths it has reached the chakra located at the navel. After ten more breaths it has reached the heart; after ten more, the larynx; and thus all the way to the top of the head, where the apprentice must visualize the flame becoming one with the masculine letter *ham*. The only stages of the process considered in this text are the five main chakras. The *svadhishtana-chakra* and *ajna-chakra* contemplated in the Tantric Hindu tradition are not mentioned. It is also possible that in the text, the exercise is used for a particular, secondary purpose, namely, for the awakening of a special form of magical warmth and for its diffusion over the whole body. This fiery fluid, called *tummo*, apparently manifests itself on the physical plane by generating an extraordinary physical heat. This heat is sometimes employed by Tibetan yogins who spend the winter season on high mountains, scantly clad (one of them was the famous magician and ascetic Milarepa) and deprived of any material protection from the freezing temperature. This exercise, though, can still be used in the context of kundalini yoga.[24]

The second exercise differs from the first only in a variation of the visualization process. Soon after imagining a flame emanating from the *muladhara-chakra*, the apprentice imagines that the letter situated on the top of the head is beginning to melt, dripping a substance that feeds the flame and that makes it rise higher and higher. Eventually the flame fills the entire sushumna up to the *sahasrara-chakra*, in which the fusion, or better, the transfiguration, of *ham* takes place.[25] The force then assumes the nature of *bodhichitta*, according to Vajrayana terminology.

In both exercises a descent follows the ascent, through the various chakras and their corresponding region until it reaches the *muladhara-chakra*. Such a process takes place simultaneously with an inversion of currents. The current of the red fluid originates and flows downward from the head; the current of the white fluid originates and flows upward from the *muladhara-chakra*.[26] I have already mentioned the idea of inversion of currents in the context of Hindu Tantrism. In yoga, pranayama aims at reversing the natural directions of prana (ascending) and apana (descending).

The type of breathing to be employed in this context is an equalized breathing from both nostrils (2t–t–2t). Conversely, a Hindu text suggests inhaling with the "sun" (pingala) and exhaling with the "moon" (ida). This text talks about the sun drinking the moon and vice versa, until a reciprocal saturation is achieved. It is, however, possible to interpret this text without a necessary reference to the serpent power. In the Tibetan texts, breathing through alternate nostrils is part of the preliminary phase of pranic saturation.

In the abovementioned Tibetan exercises, the repeated visualizations are supposed to originate a process of induction and of arousal. The images, which are prefigurations of the real process, work to make this process real. Thus, at a given moment, they are substituted with real states and with real manifestations of powers. The texts insist, however, that between the prefiguration and the experience there will always be a hiatus, and that the moment of awakening represents something discontinuous and unforeseen. The images will be transformed and act of their own initiative, as if they were animated and carried around by an extraneous force. When the process of visualization eludes the control of one who starts it, awakening is near.

The reader may recall how three chakras *(muladhara, anahata, ajna)* evoke the theme of the linga (symbol of Shiva's virility) and of the yoni, an inverted triangle symbolizing Shakti and the female genital organ. It is said that these chakras offer a particular resistance (as if they were hostile "knots") that must be overcome as breath ascends along the sushumna. In reference to everyday life, these obstacles correspond respectively to the bonds of sexual desire, of self-love, and of the intellect (especially in the form of pride). Therefore, the evoked force must overcome and transform the energies found in each of these three chakras. If the opposite thing happened, in other words, if the awakened power became attracted and finally converged onto any of these bonds, one would incur one of the greatest dangers inherent to these yogic exercises. Instead of liberation the final result would be obsession—obsession with sex, with selfishness (the opposite of this bond is a false universal and sentimental love, encompassing everything and everybody), and with a cold and detached intellectual pride (hubris).

One's whole being will end up being dominated by one of these three factors, which having escaped control are now absolutized. The correspondences that the chakras have with certain affective dispositions are not exempt from dangers. A partial awakening of a chakra could unleash the affective elements associated with it, which would thereby get out of control. Yoga teachers warn that if the preliminary discipline of purification has been neglected or found to be not energetic enough, every leftover residue will "vampirize" the awakened energy and feed demons. This belief is also found in other initiatory traditions. Hermetists talk about the "second flood" that occurs as soon as one drinks a "virgin's milk"; Mithraism talks about the onslaught of impure animals rushing to eat the "three spikes of wheat."[27] These animals, instead of blood, sprang from the side of the bull slain by Mithras. There is a teaching according to which "the ascent of the serpent power through the chakras induces the awakening and the activation of the karmic principles therein contained." This teaching warns us of the extent to which these phenomena can go. Let us also remember what has already been said concerning the samskaras and the *vasanas*, the subconscious roots whose origin often antedates the present life. These underground roots are responsible for causing the relapse into tendencies or states that were believed to be left behind once and for all, since they were removed from superficial manifestations. These roots also cause negative attitudes (greed, anger, fear, vanity, etc.) that had never been manifested before to surface. These attitudes are samskaras and *vasanas* that, all of a sudden, have become operative after having been galvanized by the new energy now circulating within one's body. This energy could also be a manifestation of ancestral samsaric forces, in other words, of the effects of remote actions and of the manifestation of entities yearning for life, with whom one stipulated obscure deals. It is easy, for somebody who does not have knowledge of these things, to become alarmed by these effects, to think that what is taking place is a spiritual regression, and therefore to abandon these "unhealthy" practices. All of this takes place within the natural logic of initiatory development, however. In this kind of development such a crisis would not take place, because the apprentice succeeded in removing every *samskara* and every samsaric residue, not only in ordinary consciousness, but in the body and in the subconscious as well.

It is also possible that the emergence or reemergence of residues will take place not in the plane of the affective life and tendencies but in the form of visions and apparitions during the yogic process, thus causing more deviations. These are so-called projections, which have been made possible through the freedom from the control of the physical senses that was acquired by the magical imagination. Once the residual or subconscious energies, which we all carry within ourselves, have been loosened, they become objectified in a world of ghosts and various deceiving apparitions, which tend to confuse the unexperienced apprentice, inducing in him a chaotic and disintegrating visionariness.

The need to be directed by a spiritual teacher is emphasized, since the teacher could help the apprentice confronted by such dangers. This help may also be invisible, since it may come through influences that do not require the physical proximity of the teacher in order to be effective. Tibetan texts call these influences "waves of gifts." In any event, in the case of reemerging and revitalizing tendencies or emotional states, or in the case of visible manifestations, in order to overcome the obstacle one should remain still, impassible, without acting or reacting. The emergence should exhaust itself, since every inner movement on the part of the yogin would give to the manifested force a grip on him and thus sweep him away. It is possible that in this way some destinies may be accomplished, even tragic and unintelligible ones, only if one follows the principle of "not resisting evil" so that everything may be expelled, consumed, and turned to ashes after the spiritual fire has burned out. These, however, are rare forms of catharsis. These forms provoke an abortive process; what has been anticipated is what would have otherwise happened in the course of one's life in more unfavorable circumstances, because of the lack of specific preparation.

In the case of apparitions and visionary phenomena ("forms of smoke," mirages, lights, etc.), the texts say that before them one must adopt a detached, though careful, attitude. One should not become interested or uninterested in one or the other; the spirit must be like that of "a child calmly looking at the walls of a temple,"[28] attentive, cautious, awaiting things to happen. This is the best way to neutralize the vampiric process and to prevent perverse kinds of vitality from feeding the apparitions. If these forms were left alone and looked upon with a calm objectivity, they would eventually wither and fade away. After that, what ensues is a state of mind that can be compared to a pure, transparent, colorless, and solid crystal, in which the experience of the tattvas is realized without distortions or darkening.

Kundalini yoga is conceived as a positive reality that can be experienced independently of one's beliefs or philosophy: "If one engages in esoteric practices, he will obtain the same results, with a scientific precision, no matter what his beliefs are." One will eventually discover "constant and invariable" elements hidden under the cover of various images, which are derived, through the subconscious, from various traditions and from the branch of one's superbiological heredity.

It is important to emphasize again that, although the yogic realizations presuppose a power of visualization identical to that of hallucinations or of hypnotic states, they develop in a state of superlucidity. Just as the hypnotizer is aware and conscious of the person being hypnotized, who "sees" what is being suggested to him, likewise the yogin is aware and conscious of his own body; the control that he exercises is very different from the kind of control one could have on a passive and extraneous subject. This is why there is a great difference between yogic feats and the spiritualistic experiences of mediums. The medium's trance is exactly the opposite of the magical state, and of the state of Shiva's presence, since it signifies regression into the subconscious and in the preconscious. In spiritualistic phenomena, the person is left at the mercy of obscure influences that move chaotically behind the natural and human reality. Every medium either already is or will fall below the human condition, while a true yogin rises above it.

· XII ·

THE DIAMOND-
THUNDERBOLT BODY

Once the yogin has acquired the capability of awakening kundalini, he attempts, through various stages of sadhana, to channel it upward through all the chakras. This process is called *urdhva-kundali* or *shat-chakra-bheda*. It is compared to the opening or blossoming of the chakras, since they are portrayed as lotus flowers, and also compared to the transformation of the profane and mundane path into a regal path, in which "there is no longer day or night," since the "sushumna swallows time."[1] In order to reach every chakra, it is a standard procedure, in yogic practice, to concentrate gradually the mental and imaginative focus on each of them, by recalling their meaning and by employing the symbols and mantras that traditional teachings attribute to them. In such a way the awakening power is properly led and induced to act.

According to the texts, those who have been successful in awakening kundalini (a selected few among all the apprentices) do not necessarily know how to bring the process to conclusion, for this is achieved by only a few. After each ascent, kundalini returns to the *muladhara-chakra*, taking again the "dormant" form, which characterizes the average human condition. Kundalini should be recaptured and reactivated in this chakra, and then led higher and higher, overcoming all obstacles blocking the access to each chakra. It is said that when kundalini reaches a given chakra, all the pranic forces that depend on it are reabsorbed into their radiant center. They also withdraw from the body and converge into the sushumna, which forms one ascending conduit in which the basic life force flows. This has a tangible physical effect. The body becomes ice cold up to the level reached by kundalini, and when the serpent power reaches the *sahasrara-chakra*, the whole motionless body becomes as cold as a cadaver, while a little warmth remains in one spot at the top of the head. This peculiar phenomenon is believed to take place only in kundalini yoga. Sometimes luminous phenomena are believed to occur, such as a radiance around the yogin's body every time he achieves various transcendent states.

When dealing with this kind of dhyana, called "purification of the elements" (*bhuta-shuddi*), I claimed that this contemplation of the transformation of the body into a quasidivine body endowed with supernatural faculties is just a mental prefiguration of what really takes place in hatha yoga. I also explained the ultimate meaning of this purification of the elements. The tattvas are experienced according to their nature, under the aegis of the "path of cessation" (*nivritti-marga*), consisting of transcendence and of pure forces exempt from any individualizing production, form, or limitation, rather than under the aegis of the "path of activity" (*pravritti-marga*), consisting in a coalescence, due to Shakti's extroverted orientation, of a substance with its modifications, of a producer with its product, of a cause with its effects. I have also shown the analogy of the ascending process along the sushumna with Mysteriosophy's "initiatory journeys." During these journeys the adept, after going through "seven heavenly spheres,"[2] and after successfully freeing himself from the influences found in each sphere, asks their respective rulers to allow him to go through, until, "possessed of his own proper power," he reaches an eighth sphere, which is a state of ultimate identification with God.

In this state the principle that was manifested as ego assumes its natural form. It is not supported by anything ("Antaeus, who derived his strength from the earth, eventually gets killed"), yet it supports everything ("Heracles has taken upon himself Atlas's burden"—according to an esoteric interpretation of the Heracles saga).[3] In the Tantric complementary belief, the *sahasrara-chakra* is described as a "place that is not a place properly speaking," in which "there is no longer a 'here' or a 'not-here,' but only the great Void, in which there is calm enlightenment, as if it were an immense ocean."[4] The Vajrayana instead sees the *sahasrara-chakra* as the seat of the great Vajradhara, the god presiding over *vajra*.

As far as the dramatic aspect of the ascent is concerned, there is an interesting parallel in the Kabbalistic doctrine of the so-called Books of the Hekhalot. The seven spheres are portrayed as seven heavenly palaces, through which one must walk before being admitted to the throne. Mounting obstacles on the way hinder the ascent. Thus it is necessary to resort to a magical seal (actually a secret "name"), which puts to flight hostile forces in every sphere. The initiate also marks himself with this seal "in order not to be swept away into fire, flames, whirlwinds, and storms." According to an interesting saying, "a fire [kundalini] emanating from his own body threatens to consume him." In this situation one is expected to stand straight, "without hands and feet" (a similar expression is "to subsist with support"). This is the same situation, according to another saying, as that of "the transformation of Enoch's flesh into burning torches," a transformation that may turn out to be destructive for those who prove not to be worthy of it.[5] According to Jewish tradition, Enoch is one of those beings who disappeared and who ascended into heaven with their bodies.

We should now consider the third "esoteric mystery" of Vajrayana tradition, which consists in the assumption into heaven of the so-called perfect or incorruptible body. This body is the equivalent of the *siddha-deha* and of the *divya-deha*, known in Hindu Tantric schools by the name of *natha-siddha*.[6] One who has brought to completion the yogic process is a *jivanmukta*, a "living liberated being." He has finally overcome the human condition and has successfully deconditioned his own being. Thus he is ready to take leave from this finite world. As I have said, a power attributed to a Tantric yogin is *iccha-mrityu*, the faculty of committing suicide through an act of the will, that is, of abandoning the body as one would toss aside a useless instrument. In any event, the yogin has already had intimations of the natural death of the organism while living in the body as a particular individual. Death appears therefore as the only opportunity to sever the last ties, this being a case of "belated liberation" (*videhamukti*). Once the yogin arrives at the "supportless abode," he will never be subject to dissolution, not even to the "great dissolution" (*mahapralaya*) in which, in conformity to the rhythm of the cosmic cycles, the entire manifestation will be reabsorbed into the principle (= the end of the world).

It is important to remember that according to the Hindu and Buddhist Tantric view, the state to be achieved is nirvana, not in

THE YOGA OF POWER

the apophatic or supernatural sense of the word, but in a sense in which the yogin is united with every power of the manifestation, and in which he is in full possession of Shakti. This view carries implications regarding the body and its use, in relationship to which the idea of "the incorruptible body" has been developed. The chakras' awakening and the occupation of their seats correspond to the occupation of occult and subtle corporeity. This implies the body's transformation or regeneration. The body is no longer experienced under tamas's aegis, that is, in a predominantly materialistic way, but under that of rajas and sattva. It should not be understood to mean that following this transformation, the outer body, as it has been studied by Western positive sciences, is no longer composed of flesh, nerves, bones, and so forth. The transformation in question regards not physical elements but their function. It signifies the I's elevation to the metaphysical plane and its union with the powers on which the physical elements depend and by which they have been made. The elements, by assuming the form of a particular being, have dissociated themselves and have become autonomous from that plane which the I now supports and rules according to its own laws. This reestablishes the "normal" condition whereby the I exists and keeps on living by depending on the physical body in which it awoke and which is now "his" (we say "his" because of the limited control it exercises over it). The new body relies on and owes its existence to the reintegrated I, and its seat is no longer the particular, ephemeral body, but the matrix or root of corporeity in general.

Thus the body is no longer "in bonds" (to use a Gnostic and Pauline expression), but becomes a "body of freedom." We also could refer to the esoteric understanding of the "resurrection of the flesh" (which has been interpreted literally by Christianity) promoted by Docetists and by Valentinians about the "apparent," nonphysical body of Christ. Also, the *siddha-kaya* and *divya-deha* of Hindu Tantrism correspond to Mahayana's theological notion of *nirmana-kaya*, which it conceives as *mayavi-rupa*. The term *nirmana-kaya* means "body produced as a result of an adequate transformation," and it designates a sort of "magical body" or "apparent body," since the attribute *mayavi* derives from *maya*. It has already been pointed out that according to some, maya is the power of the manifestation (*maya-shakti*), and that according to others, it is a power producing appearances, as well as objects that do not exist in themselves. According to Mahayana theology, those beings endowed with a buddha body, when they decide to appear and to act in a given level of existence, do not take on an ordinary body. They take on *nirmana-kaya,* which is a "projection," or an apparent body, or a magical formula, all the while remaining externally indistinguishable from a common body. Gnostic Docetism had something of this kind in mind when talking about Christ as a divine manifestation. This doctrine was obviously declared heretical from the start, since Christianity did not have the metaphysical interpretative criteria necessary to understand and to uphold this deep doctrine. Christianity also lacked an esoteric interpretation of its own tradition, according to which Christ's body, upon his resurrection, was not found in the tomb.

When a body becomes a *siddha-rupa,* in virtue of its own nature, it enjoys the possibility of "withdrawing" the form manifested in all its elements—that is, of making it disappear, as easily as "a strong man bends his stretched arm." A parallel notion is found in the previously mentioned Kabbalistic views whereby the prophet Enoch "was taken up into heaven" with his body, thus withdrawing from the manifested world without leaving his body behind. A more precise correspondence is found in the magical Taoist (*tao-chiao*) theory of the *s'i-kiai,* the "the solution of the cadaver." According to this theory, when adepts die, they do not leave their bodies behind, since they have "broken down the body," in a way similar to that in which laya yoga pursues the body's "solution" or unsealing. The Gnostic notion of "glorious body" is the equivalent of the "transformed body" notion. In Tibet, this body is called *jai-lus,* "rainbow body," and it is said that while in it, one may become invisible at will. If one agrees with the doctrinal presuppositions, there should be no difficulties in accepting this.

The theory of "conditional immortality" converges with these ideas. The premise of this theory is that in ordinary life the body constitutes the foundation of the individual's sense of identity. Thus, in order to survive death, one has to remove, in his or her body, all those conditionings that make it perishable. This was also one of alchemy's goals. We may also recall the ancient Egyptian notion of *sahu,* whereby soul and spirit, respectively the "name" and the power of an individual, are transformed and united to such an extent that, after death, they remain whole (the term *sahu* means "to stand up," "not to fall").[7] This notion is also found in Alexandrian Gnosticism and later surfaced in Western magical-initiatory traditions. According to Agrippa, neither the soul nor what he calls "twice subtle" (*eidolon*) may avoid dissolution and become immortal unless they unite with the sublime power represented by the mind, understood in this context along lines parallel with the pure Shaivist principle (*vajra-chitta*). Agrippa calls "a standing, and not a falling, soul"[8] that which has become integrated in the aforesaid fashion. Not only does "every magical virtue," namely, the capability of bringing any task to completion "by itself, stem from it without any outside help whatsoever"; but also, this is the only soul that will not experience death, along with any *eidolon* and any power or element of the organism that has undergone a similar integration. The mystical and neo-pythagorean view of the *iaugoeides*, a radiant, eternal entity enclosed in a body,[9] refers rather to the notion of subtle corporeity enclosed in the depths of the bodily structure.

These experiences are proper to the supreme achievements of hatha yoga, and they represent horizons that the overwhelming majority of human beings can perceive only from a transcendental distance. Despite this, Tantrism attributes to adepts, be they viras or divyas, thaumaturgical or paranormal powers, or siddhis. It seems that, at least theoretically, there is nothing that a yogin proficient in *shakti-sadhana* cannot do. This "power of doing anything" is susceptible to a double interpretation, in the sense of *licere* and in the sense of *posse*. The first meaning evokes antinomianism: the *siddha-yogin* can do as he pleases (he is *svecchakari*), since the merging of "three rivers" (the pingala, ida, and sushumna) renders him superior to any impurity or fault. In him there is no karma, "no sin, no virtue, no heaven, no rebirth."[10]

The terms *licere* and *posse* are somewhat interdependent. In a nondualistic worldview everything is permitted for those who can do all things, since only a higher power may set a limitation to *licere*. Tantric and Hindu metaphysics do not hold moral laws and values in the same esteem accorded to them by many Western philosophical systems. The latter tend to attribute to them an intrinsic validity, which is to say, an abstract and baseless validity. In the former, every value and law has a meaningful role to play only in a particular domain ιof conditioned existence, in which it mainly expresses the form of the power supporting it. Here it is a matter of defining the hierarchical relationship between a siddha, this power, and, generally speaking, with the degree of "deconditioning" of the siddha himself, which highlights not only strength but also the detachment characteristic of invulnerability and superiority.

It should not be assumed that every yogin devotes himself to the production of sensational and supernatural feats by employing his powers and his inviolability, thus performing wonders that ordinary people would enjoy and take pride in. The yogin truly has such powers. We also saw that in ancient texts of the Indo-Aryan tradition there is almost an ostentation in listing all the deeds that a person endowed with "knowledge" may freely perform without being blamed, since it is believed, according to antinomianism, that the spirit is beyond good and evil. At the level of pure yoga, the acquisition of powers is concomitant with the natural loss of all the instincts and passions that would induce a pashu to employ them. The yogin has no interest in such activities,[11] apart from specific circumstances. This could possibly mark a difference between the viras and the Left-Hand Path on the one hand, and the divyas on the other hand. The Tantric ideal of the coexistence of liberation and enjoyment, which consists in being open to all experiences in the world, may eventually induce a vira to pursue a practice in which he may exercise his power "beyond good and evil." Conversely, the divya, or yogin, is on too high a plane to pursue this line of conduct and to affirm himself in the domain of visible actions.

In the divya it seems that action and disregard of moral laws play a major role in overcoming ecstatic states and in effectively achieving the unconditioned. Some light may be shed on this teaching by the esoteric Islamic school of the Melewis. They distinguish three stages. In the first stage, an ecstatic beatitude is experienced by those who break free from their egos, who embrace the universe and all living beings, thus experiencing an elation that is also a deep peace. This is called a state of negative unity. In the second stage, one experiences powers, such as the ones I previously mentioned: this stage is not automatically achieved by all those who have entered the first one. It requires an affirmation and a different employment of consciousness and of the individual's will, at a point in which one no longer has desires. This is the path of pure, magical action, and if it is followed thoroughly, it leads to the third state, of positive unity. In it one finds no more ecstasies. All mystical residues have been consumed, and what remains is the realization of the supreme, unpronounceable mystery.

Those who are curious about specific powers should refer to the well-known exposition found in the third chapter of Patañjali's Yoga-Sutra, [12] since it is the general opinion that an authentic yogin, no matter what school he belongs to, is in possession of supernatural powers. More specifically, the Tantras mention these five powers: *uttakanam*, the power to avert and to repel; *vashikaranam*, the power to subdue (e.g., minds and powers); *stambhanam*, the power to arrest (e.g., a storm, render a person speechless); *vidveshanam*, the power to kindle strife and struggles; and *svastyayanam*, the power to protect, to help, and to heal. The stimulation of each chakra confers power over the corresponding elements. For instance, the awakening of the *svadisthana-chakra* makes it possible, in special circumstances, to suspend the fire's power (to render the body immune to fire) or to start a fire without those circumstances normally required to produce one. This brings us back to what was said about the mantras. In some Tibetan texts that I have often referred to, one encounters these further indications:[13] Through the earth chakra one acquires an extraordinary material strength. Through the water chakra one may acquire youthful energies, thus neutralizing the processes of aging and of organic decay ("The Water of Life"). Through the fire chakra one acquires the power of transforming and of dissolving the elements (this corresponds to the Hermetic saying *solve et coagula*). Through the air chakra one obtains the power of levitation, and also speed, both in a physical sense and in the sense of a projection of one's image in a place conjured by thought (bilocation). Through the ether chakra one will add the power to overcome the resistance of water and of the earth, that is, to be able to cross water and land. The same happens in the spiritualistic phenomena called "aport phenomena." Specific actions on the solar and lunar principles are believed to make one's body shadowless or invisible to others. The same text emphasizes the reference to a special realization that is the counterpart to these siddhis, namely, the "opening of the two spiritual doors," memory and will. They are both believed to be free of individual spatial-temporal limitations and to be open to the siddha.[14]

The Tantras go on to reaffirm the ancient Vedic-brahmanic and Buddhist belief in the siddha's superiority to all other "divinities." The siddha has power over "three worlds." No god, including Brahma, Vishnu, and Hari-Hara, can resist him. The possibility of doing as one pleases and to prevent things from happening is theoretically upheld. The siddha is "Lord of Death" (*mrityunjeya*) in the specific sense of being able to kill the body through an act of the will—the so-called *samhara-mudra*, the "act of dissolution"[15]—of not experiencing death, and of transferring one's consciousness to any chosen level of existence. A siddha, according to Milarepa,[16] "goes at will through existences as an untamed lion freely roams a mountainous region." A power often considered by Tantrism is the so-called *phowa*. On the one hand, this power consists in projecting oneself outside one's body, into "bodies" corresponding to other "abodes" or cosmic planes. On the other hand, it consists in assuming someone else's body, thus becoming the real driving force behind that person's thoughts, resolutions, and passions, which he still believe to be his. In particular, a siddha cannot lie, since his word is a word of power, which commands to reality; thus everything he says would come true. In him the fundamental Tantric motif of the unity of *bhoga* and mukti is actualized. He enjoys the dignity of *chakravarti*, of a "World Ruler,"[17] and also a freedom that cannot be experienced anywhere else. The Tantras therefore claim that there is no yoga as powerful as kundalini yoga.

In some texts, the siddhis are considered to be symptoms and supernatural proofs of all initiatory realizations, since they are not reducible to mere subjective or pseudomystical states. It is also said that these powers may represent a danger and an obstacle on the way to complete fulfillment. According to a doctrine that sees power (shakti) as the fundamental principle of the world, such a danger may arise only when the powers engender a dependency. In this case one leans on them and derives from them the meaning and purpose of one's life and self, rather than considering them with the same indifference with which ordinary people employ working tools, in which case it is obvious that through the same power one would fall back into conditioned existence, finding barred the doors of a world that "stands supportless," a world of the "naked god," wielding a royal scepter.

CONCLUSION

Aside from the ideas concerning India that feed the popular imagination (based on Gandhi, fakirs, and the like), and aside from the
prejudiced views of some Catholic thinkers (who have frequently
categorized India under the label "pantheism"), even those who
have analyzed Hindu tradition on a higher level and in greater
depth have somehow missed the point. These scholars, in fact, have
usually characterized India as the expression of a spirituality that is
essentially ascetic, contemplative, and otherworldly. According to
these scholars, India's spiritual ascetics flee the world and seek
liberation, which is obtained by being reabsorbed into formless
transcendence, or into *brahman*, as a drop of water is reabsorbed
into the ocean. After Buddhism was reduced to little more than a
humanitarian moral code and after it came to be associated with the
stereotypical concept of an evanescent nirvana,[1] the views of Vedanta
(I have already pointed out the Tantric criticisms of this darshana)
have become instrumental in shaping the current popular opinion
concerning Hindu spirituality. The views of Vedanta have been
popularized by more or less genuine contemporary epigones of
Hinduism and by various Western spiritualist and intellectual circles.
A prime example is René Guenon, an eminent exponent of integral

Conclusion

Traditionalism, who has presented Vedanta as the quintessence and most genuine expression of Hindu thought and metaphysics.[2] In relation to this, one may be inclined to believe in the thesis that claimed that Eastern civilization (by generalizing one goes from India to the whole Orient) had developed essentially under the aegis of contemplation and of world renunciation, while Western civilization had developed under the aegis of man's affirmation, action, domination, and power.

There is an element of truth in this view, which nevertheless should be criticized for its one-sidedness and incompleteness. In fact, the reader has probably recognized within the complex history of Hindu ideas and schools of thought (darshanas) the existence of a tradition that clearly contradicts the popular views concerning India's spirituality and the alleged antithesis between East and West. On the one hand, it is true that contemporary orientalists are inclined to ascribe a greater importance to Tantrism than was previously given to it. On the other hand, it has not been a long time since the West became acquainted with Tantrism. Still, it cannot be said that Tantrism has given to India its essential identity; this, however, does not mean that its role and its meaning should be overlooked.

In these final and brief considerations, I am not going to refer to Tantric yoga as such (hatha yoga and kundalini yoga) nor to its transcendent objectives, which can be achieved only by a few individuals who are exceptionally qualified and predisposed.[3] I will rather refer to those Tantric elements that are systematized in a general worldview, and in particular to Shaivism and to the Path of the Left Hand.

By referring to this worldview, I raise the danger that what I have said elsewhere[4] in an attempt to differentiate an Eastern and a Western myth (after having criticized some inconsistent and superficial views) may lose its validity. In that context I had stated, by simplification, that India was to be credited for the ideal of *liberation* and the West was to be credited for the ideal of *liberty*. On the one hand, there is the impulse to escape from the human condition in order to become reintegrated in an absolute from which we separated ourselves only to end up in a world of illusion (maya). On the other hand, there is the impulse to feel free in a world that is no longer denied, but that is rather considered as a field for action and for experiencing of all the possibilities inherent in the human condition.

Now, it is clear that with Tantrism the differentiation between liberation and liberty no longer subsists, since, as a general rule, Tantrism, in its spirit—leaving out of consideration the framework of local traditions—should be considered distinctly Western. It is more conspicuously Western than Christian soteriology, which proclaims an ideal of salvation from a world that is looked upon as a "vale of tears" and contemplates the destiny of a human nature that has been infected with sin and that stands in need of redemption.[5] In Tantrism we find a very interesting phenomenon; those ascetic techniques that were well known in India are no longer employed in order to achieve an otherworldly liberation but in order to achieve liberty within the world. These techniques are supposed to bestow on a superior human type an invulnerability that allows one to be open to every worldly experience, and that grants the power to "transform the poison into medicine." The password of Tantrism is not the incompatibility, but rather the unity, of spiritual discipline (sadhana) and enjoyment of the world (bhoga); this has led Tantrism to take issue with Vedanta's view of the world as "illusion" (maya), since Tantrism has perceived the reality of the world in terms of power, or of shakti.

We have also encountered, when examining the ethics of the Path of the Left Hand and the disciplines leading to the destruction of the human limitations (pasha), forms of anomia, or of something "beyond good and evil," which are so extreme that they make the Western supporters of the theory of the superman look like innocuous amateurs. What is significant, in this context, is the emphasis given to a dimension that these supporters of the superman totally ignore: the dimension of transcendence, or better yet, of an "immanent transcendence." We are far beyond the "blond beast" and the individualist anarchists, who are inspired by a materialistic, secular, and Darwinian worldview. We are dealing here with a liberty that, as we have seen, implies previous disciplines not dissimilar to those advocated by traditional asceticism and by a transcendent orientation. This view has almost no equivalent in the universal history of ideas.

As I have said in the Introduction, Tantrism became widespread in India around the fifth century A.D. The doctrinal formulation of its views may be dated, at latest, around 650 A.D. Between then and now have passed quite a few centuries. It is therefore interesting to notice that if we adapt the traditional Hindu doctrine of the four ages of the world (yugas), Tantrism anticipated a situation that corresponds to our modern times. Tantrism has foretold the phase of the last age (Kali Yuga), whose essential traits—those of an epoch of dissolution—can incontrovertibly be recognized in so many events and trends of our day and age. With this in mind, Tantrism has sanctioned the expiration of traditional spiritual forms that in previous epochs presupposed a different existential situation and a different human type. Tantrism also sought out new forms and new paths that might prove efficacious even in the "dark age," and it tried to implement the realization of the same ideal of other epochs, namely, the awakening and the activation of the dimension of transcendence within humankind. There is a limit to this, though. According to the Tantras, the path to be followed is that which in other times was kept secret in view of the dangers associated with it. This path is reserved only for a small minority (for the viras and the divyas): it is implicitly precluded to the masses, because, it is claimed, the majority of people living in the dark age are pashus, animal-like, conformist, limited individuals, who would not comprehend the doctrine, or who would be ruined by it, because of their lack of necessary qualifications.

We may well say that the essence of the way to be followed in the dark age is summed up in the saying "riding the tiger." I am not even dreaming of proposing Tantrism to the Western world, or of importing it here in the West, so that people may practice it in its original aspects. These aspects, as we have seen, are strictly and inseparably interwoven with local Hindu and Tibetan traditions and with the corresponding spiritual climate.[6] Nonetheless, some of Tantrism's fundamental ideas may be considered by those who wish to deal with the problems encountered in our day and age, by assuming avant-garde positions and by attempting new and valid syntheses.[7]

In my book *Cavalcare la tigre* (Riding the tiger) I have tried to indicate the existential attitudes proper to a differentiated human type who lives in an era of dissolution and in a world in which "God is dead" (naturally, this is only a theistic image typical of devotional religion, which is recently experiencing a deep crisis). In this world there are no longer any values left standing, and all the surviving traditional structures are just residues, empty shells, incapable of offering a real support and a true meaning of life. In another work of mine, *Metaphysics of Sex*, I have evaluated the potential transcendence of the sexual experience, which, as we have seen, constitutes the foundation of sexual practices of the Tantric Vamachara. In this book I wanted to indicate those elements of human sexuality that can be set against those elements that in contemporary civilization have an endemic, obsessive, and primitivist character; I also wished to set these transcendent elements against the turbid, repressed sexuality that is considered by Freudian psychoanalysis.

Having introduced the reader to a relatively unknown tradition of Hindu spirituality, very different indeed from the Vedantic and neo-Vedantic contemplative orientation; having described one of the most interesting forms of yoga, namely, kundalini yoga, in its original form, without attempting to adapt it or to popularize it, I sincerely hope that this present exposition will offer to some readers a few elements for meditation, outside the context of specialized Oriental studies and in the context of their personal problems.

BARDO:
ACTIONS AFTER DEATH

Recently the Western world has become acquainted, through various translations, with a number of Tibetan Buddhist texts concerning afterlife experiences and the opportunities afforded to the I in the postmortem state.[1] These texts are particularly interesting to Westerners because our hemisphere, which has been dominated by monotheistic beliefs, has never known such spiritual horizons. I have decided to consider these texts here, moreover, because their translators have characterized them as "works more or less Tantric."[2]

In spite of the predominantly Mahayana Buddhist worldview at the basis of such texts, the nature of the teachings contained therein is markedly Tantric. Action, in this context, takes place at the precise moment of death and even beyond death, and it aims at suspending the karmic interplay of cause and effect and eventually at realizing the unconditioned.

The Hindu tradition, both in its brahmanic and Buddhist components, had given special consideration for some long time to the notions of *jivanmukta* (one who, while still alive, rids himself of the bonds of existence) and of *videhamukta* (one who achieves the fullness of liberation only when his spirit becomes free from the hindrances of the physical body; this occurs either at death or at a later stage). Similarly to other traditions, whether religious or not, the Hindu tradition emphasizes that the way and the mental frame in which one dies have far-reaching repercussions in the next world. Tantrism alone, however, formulated a real "science of death" and emphasized the notion of "freedom of choice" toward our otherworldly destiny.

This principle does not apply to the vast majority of people, however, for whom death represents a deep crisis. The change in state that corresponds to this crisis is experienced by people as some kind of swooning or as being knocked unconscious, according to an almost mechanical connection of causes and effects called *karma* (everything one does during an earthly existence has far-reaching repercussions). This connection will determine a new conditioned existence, totally unrelated to previous lives, since there is no true personal continuity of consciousness between them all ("as a flame ignites another flame"). We may notice that one of the possible meanings of the term *pashu*—referring to the ordinary, conditioned human—is "sacrificial victim," an animal about to be sacrificed. This brings us back to the concept of *pitriyana*, which is one of the two paths to the next world considered in Hindu traditions. In this path, which most people are forced to tread, death releases personality to the ancestral forces of the stock of origin, the same way an animal is sacrificed to the gods and becomes nourishment for other lives. Thus the only thing that continues to live on is the abovementioned karmic process. This was also the case of the second path, the "path of the gods" (*devayana*). The exoteric teachings on reincarnation never put much emphasis on the deceased's freedom of choice, and understood the various changes of states leading to the great liberation to be almost automatic, or to be mere effects of a preexistent force and knowledge.[3] Conversely, the texts I have mentioned in this appendix contemplate a higher degree of indetermination and freedom, as well as the possibility of directing the supernatural processes "as a horse is led by the bridle." Through the "narrow and dangerous crossing of the *bardo*" (*bardo* designates the hereafter) the karmic determinism can be halted (even that karma which "could have led one to the deepest of all hells"), the great liberation may be achieved, and one may even create a better destiny for oneself.

As I have said before, however, these possibilities are not within everybody's reach. It is assumed, for instance, that during the earthly existence one must already have trodden a part of the

Way and sought the unconditioned, without having arrived at the end of the journey, and yet having shifted one's inner center out of samsara's reach. Therefore the texts emphasize the "great importance of having had experiences." These people, too, see death with the same traits that are seen by pashus; it befalls an individual at a given time, owing to extraneous causes. Esoteric teachings offer advice on how to prevent death from being an interruption, and how to take advantage of the postmortem states in extremis, as far as the goals pursued in life are concerned.

The starting point consists in a lucid and objective knowledge of these states. Woodroffe calls this knowledge "a traveller's guide to other worlds."[4] After giving a description of these states, the texts explain their meaning and indicate the stands one is supposed to take in each of them. These are the contents of the Bardo Thödol (the Tibetan Book of the Dead), the Egyptian Book of the Dead, and other medieval treatises, such as the *Ars moriendi*.[5] The *Bardo* belongs to the category of *terma*, namely, of "secret revelations"; it therefore has an initiatory character. According to tradition, the *Bardo* was originally composed by the sorcerer Padmasambhava, who came from northwestern India to Tibet in the eighth century. The text was hidden by him, but was recovered by his disciples in the fourteenth century. The Tibetan Book of the Dead is almost a *viaticum*; it is read by the lamas to those who are about to die, in order to prepare them for what is to come. The text contemplates the possibility that the guru may magically support a disciple's soul following the death of the body, and that he may instill in it the powers of memory and of knowledge; this obviously presupposes a highly qualified guru. These practices, however, take place within an initiatory context. After all, it was an ancient Greek teaching that "he who is not initiated is far from achieving spiritual realization; he is immersed in mud, both in this life and, more so, in the next life." Olympiodorus spoke of "two initiations: those that take place in this life, which are just a preparation, and those that take place in the heavens."[6] The latter may be associated with the experiences taking place in the *bardo* mentioned in the Tibetan Tantric texts.

At this point I do not wish to discuss the general problem of the afterlife, but simply to repeat what has already been said about the whimsical belief in reincarnation. According to the Mahayana Buddhist perspective, an individual does not constitute an indissoluble unity; on the contrary, he is an aggregate of states, stages of consciousness, and elements. The "life" that preexists birth and survives after death is not an I, but rather the central force that has determined such an aggregate. After this aggregate is dissolved, following death, the central force will determine new aggregates, according to immanent causes that were either awakened or unfulfilled in the previous existence. Such a force might be called the "samsaric I," if this were not a contradiction in terms. Buddhism calls it *santana*, which means "current," "flow," "connection of states." This force is not the transcendent Shaivist principle, because that principle is here being swept away and almost submerged by shakti, which is "desire," or a blind, irrational, and extroverted force yearning to be released. This force is not even the individual I of ordinary people, since this conscious I is only a segment or a part of this flux, and is conditioned by the contingent unity of a given aggregate.[7] At death, the aggregate dissolves and a given being gives rise to various beings ("feeds" various beings) and to various consciousness, each following its own law. What remains is the central force that creates aggregates (the *antar-bhava*, which I mentioned in Chapter IX, should be identified with it). This force can populate and become manifested in various planes of conditioned existence; it is not necessarily confined to the human or earthly plane.[8]

A case apart is that of people who have practiced initiatory disciplines or who, in very particular circumstances, have experienced an analogous "opening." These people, in addition to the samsaric force that creates aggregates, are endowed with a true I that is an extrasamsaric principle preserving its own form, even though that form is detached from all those psychic and subtle elements that determine the human condition.[9] This I still enjoys a degree of freedom and a virtual indetermination in regard to karmic laws. The Tibetan word *bardo* is made up of *bar*, which means "between," and *do*, which means "two" (*bardo*, "between the two"). Accordingly, it has been translated as "intermediate state," meaning a state between two lives. The main meaning should be instead "state between the two," referring to an uncertain state, which has not been univocally determined, almost a crossroads. This interpretation has been adopted in numerous places by the translators of the Bardo Thödol themselves. The teaching contained in this text assumes the indetermination of the postmortem states and of the moment of death confronting those who, after having followed a spiritual discipline, are capable of avoiding or of overcoming the swoon that is inherent in the change of state. These people can make a difference. These people can act and guide their own destiny. If their own strength is not sufficient to allow them immediately to reach the supreme liberation, then they are shown the means to choose a new manifestation in the conditioned world and how to avoid the worst circumstances.

The texts mostly emphasize three *bardos*, or planes of indetermination, which correspond to three hierarchically arranged crossroads or turning points: the *chikai-bardo*, the *chönyid-bardo*, and the *sidpa-bardo*. In each of these three levels is a series of doors. Those who do not succeed in the first *bardo* have the possibility to succeed in the second *bardo*; if they do not pass the test in the second bardo they still have some opportunities available to them in the third *bardo*, which concerns manifestations in more conditioned forms. It is still possible, however, that action will fail in the third *bardo* as well. This happens when the samsaric residues still retain a power strong enough to neutralize the initiatives of the I principle. In that case, the process unfolds the way it does in the pashu's case. It is therefore meaningless to talk about a true continuity, since death did not awaken a "living being." In these people we find only the aggregating samsaric force, which acts according to the aforesaid mechanism of causes and effects under the influence of desire and concupiscence. This force will eventually generate the phantasm of an individual life.

After this clarification, let us proceed to examine the various possibilities encountered in the afterlife. The core of the entire practical teaching contained in the Bardo Thödol is the Mahayanic, Tantric, and Vedantic doctrine of identity. According to this Advaita (nondualism) doctrine, there is no difference between the I and the supreme principle, since man in his essence *is* the principle, though he may not know it. Man is free when, having overcome ignorance, he implements this identity by acknowledging the metaphysical deceptiveness of everything that looks like "other," or a distinct reality, whether natural, divine, or demonic. Such an awareness consumes every bond and destroys every otherworldly spectrum. The text repeatedly encourages the deceased to hold on fast to this truth, in each phase, for here is the key to success.

As far as other details are concerned, it is necessary first to learn the "art of dying." The tired, tamasic attitude that overwhelms people before they fall asleep is extremely deleterious, and so is the anguished, resigned attitude with which most people take leave of this world. "Indomitable faith combined with supreme serenity of mind are indispensable at the moment of death."[10] The spirit must not falter; also, one should not let the mind get distracted, not even for an instant.[11] It is necessary to cut oneself free from any attach-

195

ments, and to extinguish hatred. The most important thing to do during the change of state is not so much to remember religious images as to bring to mind what one has achieved during his life, to hold on to such a memory, and to keep in mind the teachings concerning the phenomenology of the afterlife:

> Whatever the religious practices of any one may have been, whether extensive or limited, during the moments of death various misleading illusions occur; and hence this *Thödol* is indispensable. To those who have meditated much, the real Truth dawneth as soon as the body and the consciousness-principle part. The acquiring of experience while living is important: they who have then recognized the true nature of their own being, and thus have had some experience, obtain great power during the *Bardo* of the Moments of Death, when the Clear Light dawneth.[12]

The following formula is recited at one's deathbed:

> O nobly-born (so and so by name), the time hath now come for thee to seek the Path in reality. Thy breathing is about to cease. Thy *guru* hath set thee face to face before with the Clear Light; and now thou art about to experience it in its Reality in the *Bardo* state, wherein all things are like the void and cloudless sky, and the naked, spotless intellect is like unto a transparent vacuum without circumference or centre. At this moment, know thou thyself; and abide in that state. I too, at this time, am setting thee face to face.[13]

The phenomenology of death is presented in the following terms:

> Light [the whole of visible aspects of reality] subsideth and the Gross [the body, the feeling of one's body] subsideth. Thoughts subside and the Subtle [this is a reference not to the subtle form but to some subtle phenomena which take place at the time of death] subsideth.[14]

The disappearance of the sensible light and of the feeling of one's body is described in terms of a passage through those elements, which were also mentioned in ancient Mysteriosophy. In Mysteriosophy the transformations that naturally take place at death (the earth sinking into water, the water into fire, the fire into air, the air into ether) were either induced or anticipated. These are inner states in which "the perception of all material realities is totally lost and the gross element subsides." Concomitantly, the senses are reabsorbed in this order: first sight, then smell, taste, touch, and hearing. According to the Upanishads, during this state all the faculties are reabsorbed first into their roots (manas) and then into the vital force. At death the vital force, which looks like a luminous subtle force, is the vehicle employed during the ensuing changes of states by those who participated in knowledge in the course of their earthly lives.[15] After all, it is possible that the aforesaid passage through the elements is not unrelated to the lower chakras, or, in other words, that it may be related to the "sinking inward" of the human aggregate. The "air" corresponds to the chakra of the heart, and the space between it and the chakra of ether may be considered that in which, at the moment of death, the individual's crisis of consciousness takes place.

The texts indicate some internal and external signs suggesting that death is imminent. The dying person is believed to see a white light, similar to moonshine, which eventually turns reddish. The commentary to the text mentions that some Europeans have had similar experiences at their deathbed, as they pronounced words such as "Light, more light!" (*mehr Licht*—Goethe), or "The light rises!" Ignoring the nature of this phenomenon, these people may have mistaken it for a real transfiguration, instead of seeing it as a mere psychophysical change that takes place in the sense of sight at death. These changes, in the case of profane people, are accompanied by intense emotions. One experiences a kind of "smoke" that gradually obscures the mind from within. This is the moment of crisis. Those who succeed in maintaining their spirit "free from mental formations," thanks to the yogic discipline that they practiced in their lifetime, can overcome this crisis. In these people's case, the experiences of this process, as soon as they occur, will sink into a natural feeling of calm, without any sense of discontinuity. This moment is characterized by the shining of the transcendent light, which has emerged following the dissolution occurring at death. According to the text, this is supposed to happen three and a half to four days after death. Other people, on the contrary, experience swooning and slip into unconsciousness, from which they recover only after this period. During this period the secondary components and "degrees of consciousness" of the human being gradually become autonomous and go their own way, often ending up in a zone of "wandering influences." This zone is like a tank of subpersonal, inferior, or residual forces. These forces, incidentally, are responsible for causing the array of spiritualist phe-nomena.[16] It is possible that a relatively unitary form may continue to exist after death for a short period of time. This form is some kind of double, or better, an automatic and lifeless image of the deceased; it is like a second corpse—a psychic corpse—which has been left behind.

After recovering from the "swoon" (i.e., death), consciousness awakens in a state of supernatural lucidity and finally has the most decisive experience, which strikes it with the power of a thunder-bolt. This experience consists in the manifestation of the absolute, primordial light. ("From the midst of that radiance, the natural sound of reality, reverberating like a thousand thunders simulta-neously sounding, will come."[17]) This is the real test. The I should overcome all fears and be capable of identifying with this light, since it shares its metaphysical nature. Being capable of this iden-tification grants the achievement of the great liberation and the realization of the unconditioned. Every karma and every residue is eventually destroyed. The text says that this experience should be like "meeting old acquaintances." The consequence of this identifi-cation is described as the unification—as the waters of a river flow into the ocean"—of what was and was not acquired during one's lifetime (knowledge and the amount of light that had been glimpsed, the former; the totality of knowledge and of the light, the latter).

It is possible that this test may be unsuccessful, however. One may be overcome by sheer terror and lack the spiritual courage, the sacrificial élan, and the necessary lucidity for a quick identification and for a total, instantaneous rejection of avidya (transcendental ignorance). When one fails this first test, he goes from the *chikai-bardo* to the second *bardo*, called *chönyid-bardo*. On this latter plane one is faced with similar alternatives; the only difference is that these experiences are no longer free of form. One is confronted with a phantasmagorical, dreamlike world of visions and apparitions. This world is produced by an inhibited imagination, which is no longer subject to the control exercised by the senses. This imagina-tion acquires the traits of what I have called the "magical imagi-nation," which generates similar visions with an elementary inten-sity, through projections and the exteriorization of conscious and subconscious contents. *Chonyid-bardo* is a plane that offers the po-tential for liberation to those who did not perceive the uncondi-tioned in its sheer metaphysical purity, but rather perceived it in the form of a given divine figure, symbol, or cultic image. What is being decided on this plane is the capability of overcoming the mirage and of achieving a state of identification with this phantasmagorical world. This test takes place in two stages.

The unconditioned ceases to appear in its formless, thunderbolt-like nature and becomes perceivable by the senses, at first in the form of various majestic and radiant divine figures, which appear one after the other in the course of seven days. A "day" in this context has a symbolic meaning; a day could include entire epochs of human history if a temporal correlation could be established. If one does not go beyond the first apparition, the following day another apparition comes forward. As I have said, "to go beyond" means "to identify with."

The text exhorts: "Do not be weak. Do not become attached to this world." Whatever appears should be recognized as a mere reflection. The following propitiatory formula is given: "With every thought of fear or terror or awe for all apparitions set aside, may I recognize whatever visions appear as the reflections of mine own consciousness. . . . May I not fear the bands of peaceful and wrathful deities, which are mine own thought-forms."[18]

If the deceased is not up to it, no matter how much time he spent during his earthly life in contemplation or in religious devotion, he will be overtaken by fear and anguish and turn his back to the splendor and to the power of those mirages, thus failing to achieve liberation.

Since these projections make use of images that are rooted in the deepest recesses of the deceased's consciousness, the deceased will naturally be confronted by images and sights that correspond to his faith and to his tradition. Thus in the second *bardo* the Buddhist, the Christian, the Moslem, the shaman, and so forth, will all see the gods, the heavens, and the hells contemplated in their respective traditions. They become victims of an illusion thereby, since the task to be performed in this *bardo* consists in overcoming the particularism and the outwardness of these projected images, and in achieving a state of absolute self-identification typical of a reintegrated being.[19] Those who belong to the Tibetan Tantric tradition will "see" the divinities that are worshiped in the more sophisticated versions of that tradition. They will come face to face with Vajrasattva, Ratnasambhava, Amithaba, Among hasiddhi, and so on. Concerning this, the text warns about the "seven stages of ambuscade."[20] The ambuscade consists in the objective appearance of all these divinities, which is caused by the lack of spiritual power, by the inner limitation, and by the "ignorance," which has not been completely overcome, on the part of the deceased. More specifically, the text indicates the "residues" (at the time one comes before each of those divinities, in each of the seven days) that are responsible for causing fear and for inducing the deceased not to identify with them. When one is confronted by Vajrasattva he still has residues of anger and of aversion. Before Ratnasambhava one experiences residues of attachment; before Amonghasiddhi residues of envy and of hubris, and so on.

If one does not pass the test represented by this divine, calm, and radiant world, the landscape will be transformed, almost as if a kaleidoscopic mutation were taking place. When fear becomes projected and objectified into divine characters, the calm and luminous deities are followed by terrifying, wrathful, destructive, and unrestrained deities of the Kali and Shiva type—in reality they are the same deities that were previously encountered, this time with their aspect and traits altered.[21] Once again, the deceased is supposed to pass the identification test, which is now more difficult than ever. In order to pass this test, one should have practiced, during his lifetime, the cult of these deities in a Dionysian fashion. Only then will these deities be "unveiled" and one be able to realize the integration of spiritual traits that were known at the peak of earthly ritual and practices.[22] Otherwise, one will once again back up and run away in terror.

At this plane, and more so at the following plane (sidpa-bardo), the worst difficulty is caused by forces and propensities that survive the dissolution of the human aggregate, acting now in an automatic and "fatal" way. Therefore, from this phase on, it is assumed that since the distracting impulses are very powerful, this is the best time to remember the teachings contained in the Bardo Thödol. Passing the test at the second level would ensure the deceased "transfer" to the "vajra-bearers," which constitute the realms of pure forms. These realms, through the figures of the so-called dhyani-buddhas, bear a relation to the spiritual states that are realized in various phases of yogic dhyana. As a whole, these are the highest regions in the hierarchy of manifested worlds. In the Tibetan language they are called og-min (in Sanskrit akanishtha-loka), which means "no more rebirth." These are regions in which there is no longer karmic necessity to assume human rebirth. They are ruled by the following law: "Those on the Bardo plane of the same level of knowledge or spiritual development see each other"[23] where if they were on different levels, they would remain invisible to each other.

The order of apparitions goes from absolute to relative, from direct to indirect, from informal to formal. The bottom line is that the I's attitude is solely responsible for producing the transformations and the transfer of the contents of experience. The wrathful and unrestrained deities reflect and objectify the soul's apprehension and its incapability of identifying with radiant and majestic deities. Thus, unless one is capable of identifying with the gods who appear in the new experience,[24] the terror that they generate will increase and the deceased will be induced to run away. This, unfortunately, exhausts the possibilities afforded in the second crossroads, or *bardo*.

At this point one enters into the third *bardo*, the *sidpa-bardo*, and is confronted by the "alternatives concerning rebirth." Since rebirth, at this point, cannot be avoided, it is a matter of choosing a samsaric birth rather than another. Those who have also failed the test of the second *bardo* are now drawn to the most conditioned forms of all. In these people the samsaric principle, made of desire and yearning for life, has proven to be stronger than the Shaivist principle. The samsaric principle is now directing one's development in the spiritual process. Those who during their lives followed in part the esoteric path, however, now have the power, if not to suspend this process, at least to direct it. We may compare their situation to that in which a person is trapped inside an automobile running at full speed; though that person may not be able to leave the vehicle or bring it to a full stop, at least he can still control it and avoid fatal turns and crevasses. The pashu, the ordinary mortal, does not have this advantage, since at death he ceased to exist as a true center of consciousness.

This third *bardo* is characterized mainly by an intensification of the terrifying phenomenology that was present in the previous phase. One is confronted and afflicted by storms, hail, oppressive darkness, flames of entire jungles set on fire, roars of crumbling mountains, thunderbolts, the breaking of huge ocean waves, furies and demons, deserted landscapes, endless deserts, and so on. These are all mirages, reflections, specters, and hallucinations created by spiritual impulses, or better, by the interplay of karmic forces, which have taken the upper hand and which attempt to lead one's consciousness (by way of deception and intimidation) toward a given womb door. The process unfolds in such a fashion as to make a given womb door look like a safe haven. The unsuspecting spirit, lacking self-control, is tricked into it. The texts also mention three invisible precipices, which open wide before those who run away. The precipices, whose colors are white, red, and black, correspond to the three species of births, namely, the three forms of inferior samsaric manifestations.

The second characteristic of this third *bardo* is the increasing awareness of being dead, accompanied by a strong desire to live again—the form to which one is attached is a "desire body"[25]—and by the perception of objects and beings living on various planes of existence. One's desire and reactions before the terrifying phantasmagoria must be dominated in this last series of otherworldly experiences. It is said that mind and memory here become distinctly lucid—even in those in which they were obfuscated and obtuse—and that the "desire body" acquires the quality of a magical body, since it may achieve whatever it conceives and yearns for. Because of the samsaric element, deceiving perspectives may arise, making attractive and desirable that which is not, and vice versa. The text exhorts one to be aware of the "opposition,"[26] namely, of the presence of forces that are hostile to enlightenment. These may be characterized as counterinitiatory forces, which tend to dominate the very root of the samsaric element.

"The boundary line between going upwards or going downwards is here now," the text adds.[27] Also: "Abandoning all feelings of attraction and repulsion, with memory's heedfulness restraining the roving tendencies of the mind, apply thyself to the choosing of the womb-door."[28]

Various techniques are indicated in order to avoid the choice of unfavorable wombs, which may turn out to be fatal to some people. The first technique is the method employed in the second *bardo*. One must come to realize that all apparitions are mere hallucinations and that, since the nature of one's being is emptiness, *(shunyata),* there is nothing to be feared, or nothing that threatening beings and wild forces can possibly hold on to. One must also think that these forces—including various demons, hells, heavenly judges, and so on—are just unreal forms, of the nature of echoes, dreams, mirages, or apparitions caused by magic. By inhibiting every irrational spiritual impulse, the automatic development of the karmic process is thus prevented.[29]

Concerning the entrance into a human womb, the Tibetan teachings almost resemble Freudian psychoanalysis. The being who yearns for a new life sees various couples engaging in the act of intercourse:

If to be born as a male, attraction towards the mother and repulsion towards the father, and if to be born as a female, attraction towards the father and repulsion towards the mother, together with a feeling of jealousy [for one or the other] which ariseth, will dawn upon thee.[30]

Through these feelings of attraction and repulsion, what takes place is the embodiment of a new embryo, whose gender depends on an identification with either the man or the woman. One therefore should inhibit any desire or personal preference. "Holding the mind one-pointedly upon the resolution," one must be on guard in order to prevent the arising of any feeling of desire or repulsion usually induced by the supersensible vision.

Another method has the same structure as the contemplative techniques that precede the Tantric sexual practices. One can avoid being drawn to a couple engaged in sexual intercourse by visualizing man as a male deity and woman as his Shakti or as the Great Mother.[31] A third method consists in exorcising visualizations, a method that resembles some of the Jesuit spiritual exercises. When one experiences the tormenting fury of the elements and of demons, the thing to do is to immediately visualize a magical divinity of one's choice (Heruka, Hayagriva, or Vajrapani) as a powerful, perfect, and mighty god, capable of terrifying enemy forces and various ghosts. In this way the process is halted once again, thus allowing one freely to choose the womb door. "Since thou now possessest a slender supernatural power of foreknowledge, all the places of birth will be known to thee, one after another. Choose accordingly."[32]

Keeping in mind that a good womb-door may look unattractive, one should avoid any possible inclination or feeling of revulsion, so as not to be deceived. Even though a womb may appear good, do not be attracted; if it appear bad, have no repulsion towards it. To be free from repulsion and attraction, or from the wish to take or to avoid, to enter in the mood of complete impartiality, is the most profound of arts. Excepting only for the few who have had some practical experience [in psychic development], it is difficult to get rid of the remnants of the disease of evil propensities.[33]

Here, too, it is clear that the capability of mastering one's destiny in the afterlife implies the presence, in the postmortem states, of the yogic characteristics of apathy, detachment, and a cold and majestic magic quality. It must be possible to evoke and to actualize these characteristics in order to be in complete control of oneself during this succession of free forces and images, just like somebody who keeps calm and in control of the situation under dangerous circumstances in order to choose the best course of action. Also, it helps to remember one's "secret name, which was received at the moment of initiation"; in fact, one appears before the "Lord of Death" with that particular name.

In the third *bardo* (the last of the three possible postmortem indeterminate phases), it is possible to achieve, if not liberation, at least a certain degree of freedom in the conditioned world. The choice that determines whether one is to continue or to complete the "great work" in the next existence is contingent on the degree of "recollection" that has been preserved. This case is similar to that of an individual who already enjoys privileged predispositions toward what I have called "natural dignity," and who is more or less aware of his prenatal background.

A case apart is that of those who take on a body and reappear in the human world of their own free will and not because they have missed the opportunity in the three *bardos* by failing to pass the afterlife tests, or on the basis of various determinisms. Generally speaking, these "descents" are mostly associated to a specific visible or invisible mission. In some extreme cases, one takes on a *nirmana-kaya* as a *mayavi-rupa* (see Chapter XII). In these cases what becomes manifest is not a particular individuality, but rather a force from above. The Tibetan doctrine of the so-called *tulku* claims that this force may be "reborn" in several beings at the same time, in the same way that a flame can light several wicks. The initiatory, regal, and pontifical *pluralis maiestatis* "We" may be a distant and obscure reference to this.

Those who share the metaphysical views of Mahayana Buddhism, which takes the doctrine of nonduality (Advaita) to the extreme consequence of abolishing the distinction between nirvana and samsara, will consider these views to be relative as well.

> The Mind is the Cosmos. To the Enlightened One, this apparent duality has no existence, since neither *samsara* nor *nirvana* are two things apart from individualism, but merely two aspects of One, which is the All-Knowledge, All-Wisdom. Hence, as the texts teach, *samsara* and *nirvana* are, in this occult sense, said to be inseparable. Duality is present in appearance, but not in essence.[34]

✦ Appendix Two ✦

SHAKTISM AND
THE WORSHIPERS OF LOVE

Some aspects of Hindu Shaktism, especially in the evocative dimension, are somewhat similar to the inner, esoteric aspects of medieval European movements such as the "Worshipers of Love," to which the celebrated Italian poet Dante Alighieri belonged. I think it is worthwhile to mention some of these analogies. I have dealt at greater length with the initiatory experiences of the Worshipers of Love in another work of mine.[1]

We are all familiar with the role that women played in troubadour songs and chivalric literature, in the "Courts of Love," and in the works of numerous poets who called themselves Worshipers of Love. In the love stories of contemporary literature, however, the esoterism that is partially present in it has been ignored and at times underdeveloped, owing to the academic and profane mentality of the authors. The emphasis that writers such as Aroux and G. Rossetti placed on the hidden meaning of several poems and on their multivalent language went unheeded. In Italy a fundamental work such as Luigi Valli's *Dante e il linguaggio segreto dei fedeli d'amore*, written with a critical and analytical precision, has been totally ignored by the academic establishment.

The main point I am trying to make is as follows: It cannot be denied that there are cases in which the women alluded to in this kind of literature, which was bent on exalting and celebrating them, were "sublimations," personified allegorical figures, and theological abstractions. No matter what name these women had, or what they looked like, they were all representations of the one archetypal woman, whose meaning and function, generally speaking, correspond to the Tantric Shakti's, or to the initiatory/initiating woman's. If these women really existed, they were celebrated not by virtue of their historical existence, but only because they somehow incorporated or served as the foundation of that Woman, who was conceived as the enlightening principle ("Holy Wisdom") of the Worshiper of Love's transcendent vivification and immortality. The analogy, however, must be circumscribed to what I have called the platonic plane, or to the "subtle" employment of women in Tantrism. I do not think that the West made much progress on this line. For one thing, women in the West were never employed in rituals such as the Tantric *panchatattva*, in the course of which one has sex with a woman; this woman has been transformed into Shakti, with the purpose of evoking and of awakening in her the "absolute woman."

Love has a double meaning in what I repute to be the most significative aspects of that literature. The first meaning concerns immortality and the "deathless" element. This was clearly expounded by Jacques de Baisieux, who interpreted the word *amor* as *a-mors*, literally "deathless." This author went as far as to associate *amor* with the Hindu *amrita*, the "deathless" nectar (ambrosia), which is spoken of in various Hindu texts. The second meaning deals with the rapture that "woman" kindles in man. This rapture is believed to have ecstatic effects, leading to the experience of immortality, and to the achievement of well-being (when "well-being" is understood as salvation, we may associate this term to the Western equivalent of the Hindu notion of liberation). According to the first meaning, we may see how in the literary productions of the Worshipers of Love, personified Love has Shaivist traits, which are radically different from those sentimental and stereotypical images of various Cupids armed with bow and arrows.

This is also the case in Dante's works. Dante calls Love "glorious Lord"[2] and puts these words in his mouth: "I am as the center of a circle, to which the parts of the circumference stand in equal relation; but thou not so" *(La vita nuova* [The New Life] 12:22). "Love," unlike ordinary men, is characterized by "centrality," stability, and immutability. In Tantrism these characteristics are attributed to the Shaivist principle rather than to the Shaktic principle.

Thus Love may look scary and even terrifying to an ephemeral and transient being, precisely because of its centrality and transcendence. Love sends "woman" forward and even offers her up to the initiatory experience. A word of caution is in order, however: this is a risky experience, bordering on death, since the alternative is either to become awakened or to receive a deadly blow. This is why Love says, "Flee if to perish be irksome to thee" (15:22). Dante himself says, "suddenly Love appeared to me, the memory of whose being maketh me shudder" (3:58–59). In one particular vision, Love appears "in the figure of a lord of fearful aspect" (3:20), which is the inner ruler, and says: "I am thy Lord." Dante goes on to say:

> In his arms methought I saw one sleeping, *naked*, save that she seemed to me wrapped lightly in a crimson drapery; whom gazing at very intently, I knew to be the *lady of the salutation*, who the day before had deigned to salute me. And in one of his hands methought he held a thing that was all aflame; and methought he said to me these words: *Vide Cor tuum* [Behold thy heart!]."[3]

The woman's "salutation," in the literature of the Worshipers of Love, has a coded meaning based on the double meaning of the terms *salutation* and *salvation*.[4] It is said: "Let him who merits not salvation [liberation], never hope to have her company [Beatrice's or the woman's]" (8:54). The woman who extends the salutation is the same woman who bestows salvation, or better, who propitiates a crisis and an experience that leads to salvation. Thus Dante speaks of the effects of a salutation, that often go far beyond his own strength. After all, the sight of the woman almost causes one to die. Dante says about this: "I have set my feet in that region of life beyond which one cannot go with intent to return" (14:41). And more specifically: "And whoso should endure to stay and behold her, would become a noble thing or else would die: and when she findeth one worthy to behold her, he proveth her virtue; for this befalleth him, that she giveth him salutation."[5]

The general theme of the Worshipers of Love is that, as in initatory Shaktism, "love" and "woman" actualize something that is found in a man in potency or dormancy. This theme corresponds, in Aristotle's philosophy, to the "potential intellect" (since it is not a given, but exists only as a possibility) and, in Tantrism, to the Shaivist element, which prior to intercourse with the "woman" is inactive and useless. Once this element is awakened, it prevails over anything that is human and samsaric. At the opening of *The*

New Life Dante mentions the experience of "contact." He talks about the apparition of the "glorious lady of my mind," who "was called Beatrice by many who did not know what to call her" (II, 4; in other words, they did not know what this experience consisted of). This marks the beginning of a radical transformation of the human being: At that point I verily declare that the vital spirit which dwelleth *in the most secret chamber of the heart* [i.e., the atman, which the Upanishads localize in precisely the same spot, conceived as individual principle = *jivatma*] began to tremble so mightily that it was horribly apparent in the least of my pulses, and trembling, it said these words: "*Behold a god stronger than I, who coming shall rule over me.*"[6]

What is announced is the awakening of the inner ruler, who is "the lord on the throne." The "animal spirit," which is here equated with the vital principle, is astonished at the incipient transformation: "Now has appeared your bliss." Finally, the "natural spirit," which could be equated with the samsaric nature, begins to weep and finally says: "Alas, wretched, because often from now on I shall be hindered." In other words, it realizes that it will no longer control the Worshiper of Love's being. Dante goes on to say: "From thenceforth I say that Love held lordship over my soul, which was early bounden unto him."

In the previously mentioned passage the "woman" is related to the "knowledge of the heart," and to something that is "all aflame," as if it were the center of a magic, life-giving fire. All of this helps us to appreciate the deepest meaning of the title Dante gave to his book, namely, *The New Life*. Even the sleeping woman, wrapped up in a crimson drapery, may be a highly symbolic figure. She could be equated with the "woman" found in the bloodstream, who induces the Tantric divya to claim that he has no need for external women.

The initiatory experience of the Worshipers of Love and of analogous Western movements, as well as of the Shaktic adept, is based on these points. Love induces a deep crisis, and it awakens a power that almost "kills" the subject, thus activating a superior principle hidden in man. The "woman," in turn, generates a new being, causing a new hierarchy of the powers of human nature, to be formed; this is "salvation," and the principle of a new life.

It is obviously difficult to determine in which practical existential situations all these plans have been successfully implemented. In such cases what must have taken place is a kind of evocation of and a contact with the supersensous, "subtle" plane, although a real woman may actually have facilitated the contact. Probably, as in certain aspects of Tantric practice, specific states may have been induced. In these states an exasperated desire, which was rendered spiritual through the inhibition of every material discharge, eventually consumed itself by flowing into a superior experience. This has led some to talk about the "mystery" of medieval platonic love. It is important to show another similarity. In the Tantric ritual a man, for a long period, which has been divided into three phases, must spend the nights in the same room with the young woman he has appointed to be his Shakti, and must even sleep with her, without possessing her physically. This, I think, represents the preliminary level of the "subtle intercourse." Not among the Worshipers of Love, but among the knights dedicated to the cult of the "woman," the ultimate trial, called *asag*, consisted in spending a night in bed with the woman totally naked, without any sexual act; this was done not to implement chastity, but to increase the desire for her.

GLOSSARY

ahamkara Lit. "I-maker"; the attribution of perceptions, forms, and properties to the ego; the ego sense.

antahkarana Lit. "inner instrument"; refers to the psychological powers that determine the specific experience of a conditioned being.

antahrmukhi, antarmukha Lit. "looking inward" (inwardly cognitive); refers to introversion, as opposed to *bhahirmukhi*, "looking outward" (outwardly cognitive), which refers to extroversion. In Tantric metaphysics the latter term denotes the unfolding of the manifestation (descending phase), while *antahrmukhi* consists in the reabsorption of the manifestation (ascending phase) into the supreme principle.

apana One of the principal currents of the human being's life force.

asana A ritual bodily posture assumed in Yoga. The term is often synonymous with *mudra*.

atman In the Upanishadic metaphysical tradition, the transcendental Self, which is identified with the supreme principle. In Tantrism it denotes the Shaivist principle of being.

avidya Lit. "nescience"; spiritual ignorance.

bhahirmukhi See *antahrmukhi*.

bhoga Enjoyment, use of something. The opposite of renunciation.

bija Seeds or roots; refers especially to words of power, or *mantras*.

bindu Lit. "dot"; in metaphysics it designates the level where the powers of the manifestation are gathered in one supreme unity, called *parabindu*, "supreme source." In Tantric usage it also denotes semen.

buddhi The highest or deepest aspect of the human psyche. Free from any particular determination, it is the most refined as well as the simplest form of existence.

chakra Lit. "wheel" or "disk"; used to describe the centers of occult corporeity; also designates a circle of initiates practicing collective rituals.

chidrupini-shakti Shakti assuming Shiva's nature and conscious form.

chitta Denotes mind in general, or consciousness.

deva, devata Deity.

devi Goddess.

dharma A term with many meanings: e.g., law, truth, a being's nature.

dhyana Meditation; contemplation; a phase in dhyana yoga.

divya Divine; in Tantrism it refers to people characterized by *sattva-guna*.

ekagrata The mind's power to focus attention on something; to be single-minded.

guna One of the three fundamental aspects of power displayed in manifestation. See pages 40–41.

guru Spiritual teacher.

hamsah The vital principle in its particular relationship with breath and *prana*. The term has several other meanings.

ida One of *prana's* channels of occult corporeity; it has a feminine and "lunar" character (cf. *pingala, sushumna*).

Ishvara Lit."lord"; God, theistically conceived. In Tantric metaphysics Ishvara is thought of as *bindu*.

japa Recitation of a formula or *mantra*.

jiva The individual as a living being.

jnana Knowledge, wisdom. Jnana yoga follows the path of contemplative knowledge.

Kali In Hindu mythology she is Shiva's bride; she also personifies Shiva's destructive aspect.

Kali Yuga The "dark age," the last of the four ages in the cosmic cycle.

kama Desire, pleasure.

karana, karya Cause and effect, respectively .

karma Lit. "action"; more specifically, the immanent law of cause and effect.

kaula Member of a *kula;* a follower of the Tantric spiritual path of the

Kaula sect. The term may also designate a "follower of the Goddess" (*kaulini* = *kundalini*).

kaya Lit. "body"; in a general sense, the term means "way of being" and even "seat." Three bodies are recognized: a causing body, a subtle body, and a material body, the latter being the body in the ordinary sense of the word.

kula The feminine aspect of the absolute; family; flock.

kundalini The form in which the primordial shakti is present in one's occult corporeity; the "serpent power," portrayed as a coiled snake, which alludes to its potential state preceding its awakening.

linga The phallus; as Shiva's symbol, it denotes not only sexuality but also the spiritual virility manifested in ascetic practices and in yoga.

mahabhutas The "great elements," similar to the elements constituting Spinoza's *natura naturans*. The elements in the physical world (earth, fire, air, water, ether) are their manifestations.

Mahayana One of the two major divisions of Buddhism; it has metaphysical overtones, has been influenced by Vedanta, and has initiatory elements.

maithuna Sexual intercourse.

manas Lit. "mind"; the lower mind, which organizes the information received from the senses.

mantra Liturgical formula; in Tantrism, a "word of power"; the "name" of things and of entities, encapsulated in a magical operative formula.

maya A principle through which one experiences the world as a self-subsistent reality, or as an ontological non-I; that experience, however, is an illusion caused by ignorance (*avidya*). In Tantrism the term designates a power (*maya-shakti*) that is in turn identified with the demiurgic power of the supreme principle.

mudra A synonym for *asana*, a ritual bodily posture or gesture; one of the five substances used in the secret ritual; one of the names by which young women devoted to Tantric sexual practices are called.

mukti, moksha Liberation, release; the deconditioning of being.

nadi One of the channels in which *prana* circulates in the body.

nyasa Sacramental Tantric ritual in which one's body parts are gradually assimilated to one's chosen deity.

panchatattva Lit. "five substances"; the name given to the so-called secret ritual of the Left-Hand Path, which involves the employment of intoxicating beverages and the inclusion of women.

pasha Ties, bonds.

pashu One who is subject to *pasha*; an animal-nature individual. In Tantric usage, the term refers to ordinary people who are enslaved to moral and religious precepts, which they follow in a conformist way while ignoring their deepest meaning.

pingala One of the three primary channels of the life force *(prana)* found in the occult corporeity. It has a masculine and a "solar" character (cf. *ida, sushumna*).

prajna A synonym for *dhyana;* wisdom, knowledge.

prakriti In the Sankhya system *prakriti* designates nature, as opposed to the purely spiritual principle *(purusha)*. In Tantrism it is associated with Shakti, Shiva's counterpart.

prana Lit. "life"; a transcendental life force, related to breath.

pranayama The body of yogic techniques based on breath control.

purusha In the Sankhya system *purusha* is the male, immutable, bright principle, which in Tantrism is identified with Shiva.

rajas One of the three *gunas.* See pages 40–41.

sadhana Means of realization; spiritual path, discipline.

samadhi The last phase in classic yoga.

samsara The phenomenal, ever-changing, contingent world; the conditioned existence.

samyama The complex of mental operations that in yoga lead to the apprehension of the reality behind symbols, phenomena, etc.

sattva One of the three *gunas.* See page 40.

shastra Textbook, treatise employed by a given school.

Shiva The personification of the static, luminous, and masculine form of the divine, which is opposed to Shakti's feminine, dynamic, and life-giving form; Shiva corresponds to Sankhya's *purusha.*

shunya, shunyata The metaphysical void, synonymous with transcendence (as opposed to fullness, which corresponds to the manifested reality).

siddha Adept; a designation of Tantric initiates.

siddhi Accomplishment, realization; magical powers.

sukha Joy, pleasure.

sushumna The channel of occult corporeity through which *kundalini* ascends after having been awakened (cf. *ida, pingala*).

tamas One of the three *gunas.* See page 40.

tanmatras The hyperphysical powers that determine and shape reality.

tattvas Principles; in speculative Tantrism, the levels in which Shakti's manifestation is articulated.

vada Doctrine.

vajra "Diamond" and "thunderbolt"; the term is employed mainly in Mahayana Buddhism. A scepter (Tib. *dorje*), which in turn symbolizes a thunderbolt, used in magical ceremonies.

Vajrayana Lit. "Diamond vehicle"; Tibetan Buddhist Tantrism.

Vamachara Lit. "Left-Hand Path"; a school of Tantric Shaivism.

vayu The five main pranic currents in the human body.

vidya Knowledge; in Tantric esoteric usage, a woman participating in the sexual practices.

viparita-maithuna "Inverse" sexual intercourse, in which the woman moves on top of the man.

vira Lit. "hero"; special category of Tantric initiates characterized by manly qualities, such as courage and propensity to engage in radical Dionysian rituals; a synonym for *kaula*.

virya The masculine strength required in *sadhana* and in yoga.

vrittis Modifications of mental elements; the fluctuations of consciousness. In Hindu cosmology, the modifications assumed by the supreme principle in its manifestation.

yantra A graphic symbol.

yogin A male practitioner of yoga.

yogini A female practitioner of yoga; a female deity, a yogin's spouse, and even Shakti herself.

ENDNOTES

Translator's Introduction

1. Thomas Sheehan, "Myth and Violence: the Fascism of Julius Evola and Alain de Benoist," *Social Research* 48 (Spring 1981): 45–73; idem, *"Diventare Dio:* Julius Evola and the Metaphysics of Fascism," *Stanford Italian Review* 6 (1986): 279–82. Richard Drake, "Julius Evola and the Ideological Origins of the Radical Right in Contemporary Italy," in *Political Violence and Terror: Motifs and Motivations,* ed. Peter Merkl (Berkeley and Los Angeles: University of California Press, 1986), 61–89; idem, "Julius Evola, Radical Fascism, and the Lateran Accords," *Catholic Historical Review* 74 (1988): 403-19; idem, "The Children of the Sun," in *The Revolutionary Mystique and Terrorism in Contemporary Italy* (Bloomington: Indiana University Press, 1989).

2. The essays were published in 1973 under the title *Meditazioni delle vette* [Meditations on the peaks] (La Spezia: Edizioni del Tridente, 3d. ed., 1986).

3. "In this state, life, almost like heat generating light, becomes free and other than itself. This is not meant in the sense of the annihilation of one's individuality in a sort of mystical union, but in the sense of a self-transcending act of affirmation. Following this act, feelings such as anxi-

ety, constant yearning, concupiscence, and restlessness, which are still found in those who seek refuge in faith or in other human values, finally give way to a state of calm and self-control" *(Meditazioni delle vette,* 25).

4. Evola still advocated the privilege of taking one's own life both in his *Etica aria* [Aryan ethics] and in *La dottrina del risveglio* [The Doctrine of the Awakening.]

5. Most of Evola's books have been translated into French, Spanish, and German. The only works by Evola that so far have been translated into English are *Eros and the Mysteries of Love,* (Rochester, Vt.: Inner Traditions, 1983) and *The Doctrine of the Awakening,* trans. E. Mutton (London: Luzac, 1951), and *The Hermetic Tradition,* trans E. Rehmus, (Rochester, Vt.: Inner Traditions, 1993).

6. "I have always maintained myself free of any ties to the society in which I live, since I never had professional ambitions or inclinations for a family life or for a sentimental routine" *(Il cammino del cinabro* [The cinnabar's journey] [Milan: Scheiwiller, 1972], 15).

7. In 1961 Evola wrote again about philosophy in his *Cavalcare la tigre* [Riding the tiger] (Milan: Scheiwiller, 1961), in which he laid existentialism, relativism, and nihilism on the Procustean bed of his worldview.

8. Evola, however, accused Stirner of being trapped in the snares of anarchical individualism and of lacking transcendental reference points capable of exercising a regenerating part in the individual's development.

9. *Il cammino del cinabro,* 39.

10. C. G. Jung, *Psychology and Alchemy* (Princeton, N.J.: Princeton University Press, 1968), 228, 242.

11. In 1964 he wrote *Il fascismo: Saggio di una analisi critica dal punto di vista della destra.* [Fascism: A critical essay from the viewpoint of the right].

12. As in the case of the signing of the Concordat with the Vatican and of the "demographic campaign" willed by Mussolini to increase the population.

13. "It is legitimate to seek dangers and risks, not so much out of an *amor fati,* but rather as a way to question destiny in order to find out more about oneself and one's prenatal will" *(Il cammino del cinabro,* 206). It was his innermost conviction that nothing can happen to us outside the self-made destiny raised by our actions according to the retributive karmic laws.

14. Marguerite Yourcenar, *Le temps, ce grand sculpteur* (Paris: Gallimard, 1983), 201.

15. Ibid., 204.

16. Evola was called "a guru of the counterculture Right," or "the Marcuse of right-wing culture."

17. Majjhima-Nikaya 139.

18. Sheehan, "Myth and Violence," 54.

19. In Mozart's *Don Giovanni* the statue of the murdered *commendatore* comes to life in the form of a stone guest. Invited to dinner by Don Giovanni, he replies: "Those who have tasted the food of angels no longer desire the food of mortal men."

Endnotes

CHAPTER 1

1. I wrote at greater length about this doctrine in my *Rivolta contro il mondo moderno*. This doctrine, upheld by Hesiod in ancient Western civilization and corresponding to that formulated by various Hindu texts, describes the main phases of the degenerative process at work in history.

2. Mahanirvana-Tantra 2:14–15. This text explicitly states that the teaching proper to the first age (Satya Yuga) was that of shruti, or the Veda; of the second age (Treta Yuga), smriti; of the third age (Dvapara), Puranas; of the last age (Kali Yuga), Tantras and Agamas.

3. Its decisive role is emphasized, among other texts, in the Shiva-Samhita 2 and 4:9.

4. Julius Evola, *The Doctrine of the Awakening*, trans. E. Mutton (London: Luzac, 1951).

5. Tantrattva 1:27.

6. Sir John Woodroofe, *Shakti and Shakta*, 5th ed. (Madras: Ganesh, 1959), 18.

7. K. Dawa-Sampdup, commentary to the *Shricakrasambhara-Tantra*, ed. Arthur Avalon (London and Calcutta, 1919), 23.

8. Hatha-Yoga-Pradipika 1:66.

9. Mahanirvana-Tantra 4:80, 8:203. In an interesting parallelism, a late Orphic-Pythagorean text considers, besides the four ages indicated by Hesiod and corresponding to the Hindu yugas, a further age, under the aegis of Dionysius. Dionysius was considered, in one of his main aspects also emphasized in Left-Hand Tantrism, to be a god similar to Shiva.

10. Kularnava-Tantra 1:23; Mahanirvana-Tantra 4:39: "Where there is abundance of enjoyment, of what use is it to speak of yoga, and where there is yoga, there is no enjoyment, but the kaula enjoys both."

11. A concomitant phenomenon in the Buddhist Far East was the advent of Amidism. In my *L'arco e la clava* (Milan, 1967), chapter 15, I exposed the ideal locus of such trends, as well as the absurd claim that they represent a higher form of spirituality and a superior phase in the evolution of religious thought, since they are themselves affected by the negative climate proper of the "dark age." The same applies foremost to Christianity, a religion typical of the Kali Yuga.

12. According to De la Valée Poussin (*Bouddhisme: Etudes et matériaux*, [Paris, 1898], 148, in Tantric Buddhism, the so-called Vajrayana, the Absolute ceases to be an ecstatic experience in order to become something that those who have achieved enlightenment may freely control. As far as the meaning of *Vajrayana* is concerned, Arthur Avalon remarked: "As the diamond is hard and indestructible, and as the thunderbolt is powerful and irresistible, likewise the term *vajra* is used to describe that which is stable, permanent, indestructible, and powerful." A special kind of scepter used during magical rituals and ceremonies symbolizes the *vajra* and is even called by the same word.

13. Arthur Avalon edited a group of Tantric texts, ten volumes in all, besides the Mahanirvana-Tantra. He also authored *Shakti and Shakta* (3d ed.,

London and Madras, 1928), *The Serpent Power* (London, 1925), *The Garland of Letters* (Madras, 1922), *Hymns to the Goddess* (London, 1913), *The World as Power* (London, 1930), and various minor works. Concerning Kashmir Tantrism, see the works and translations by L. Silburn.

14. Mainly the two books *Tibetan Yoga and Secret Doctrines* (London, 1935) and *The Tibetan Book of the Dead* (London, 1927).

CHAPTER II

1. Woodroffe, *Shakti and Shakta*, 2d ed., 14.
2. Ibid., 69.
3. Ibid., 3d ed., 19.
4. After all, our contemporaries were surprised to discover that in some traditional societies some elements characteristic of modern scientific knowledge, such as complex algebraic calculations, were also known. Those societies merely arrived at them just through different methods.
5. Tantrattva 1:24, 227, 2:34.
6. Kulachundamani-Tantra 1:24–25.
7. Isha-Upanishad 9.
8. Augustine, *In Psalmum CXXXIV*, 4: "He is such that in relation to Him all created things are not. When they are not referred to Him, they are [this is illusory existence, maya]; when referred to Him, they are not."
9. Tantrattva 1, chapter 4 *passim.*, pp. 224ff.
10. Jnanenralal Majumdar, introduction to Isa Upanishad, ed. Arthur Avalon (London, 1918), 7.
11. Source not given in the original edition of this book.

CHAPTER III

1. Woodroffe, *Shakti and Shakta*, 2d ed., 164.
2. In a text called *Mahakala-Samhita*, it is written: "Thou art neither male nor female nor neuter. Thou art inconceivable, an unmeasurable power, and the being of all that exists. Void of all duality, thou art the supreme *brahman*, attainable in illumination alone"(Woodroffe, *Shakti and Shakta*, 26).
3. Mahanirvana-Tantra 5:1.
4. Tantrattva 2:355.
5. Woodroffe, *Hymns to the Goddess*, 3d ed. (Madras: Ganesh, 1964), 4.
6. Ibid., 128.
7. Tantrasara 178.
8. Mahanirvana-Tantra 4:14.
9. Tantrattva 1:194.
10. "The acts of creation are for the Lord merely His play and are not ne-

cessitated" (J. Woodroffe, *Kamakala-vilasa*, 3d ed. [Madras: Ganesh, 1961], 2.

11. This term is usually translated as "philosophical system," but the literal meaning is "what can be seen from a given perspective." Generally speaking, the main Hindu "philosophies" are not isolated and closed systems, but rather expressions of one traditional doctrine, and they vary precisely according to the perspective that one adopts.
12. Maitri-Upanishad 3:2.
13. Tantrattva 2:46–47.
14. Ibid., 2:27.
15. Kamakalavilasa 7, 8.
16. Ibid., 9, 10.
17. Tantrattva 1:312.
18. Mahanirvana-Tantra 4:34.
19. Mandukya-Upanishad 5–7. See also Maitri-Upanishad 7:11:7–8.
20. P. Deussen, *Sechzig Upanishaden*, 3d ed. (Leipzig, 1921), 2:8, 9.
21. "In this dualistic world, with all its variety of names and forms, father, mother, brother, sister, wife, son, daughter, you and I, nonmoving and moving things, insects, flies, and the other names and forms that we see, are all only the *parabrahman* manifesting itself in different forms, such forms being due to change by maya, and in reality, nothing but a manifestation of *parabrahman*" (Tantrattva 1:276).
22. We read in the Kularnava-Tantra (9:47): "Jiva is Shiva and Shiva is Jiva, the only difference being that one is bound, the other is not."
23. Tantrattva 1:83–87.

Chapter IV

1. René Guenon, *Man and His Becoming According to the Vedanta*, trans. Charles Whitby (London: Rider, 1928), 72.
2. Kamakalavilasa 36.
3. Tantraloka-Ahnika 3.
4. Prapanchasara-Tantra, 1:4.
5. Isha-Upanishad 9, 10.
6. Concerning the *kankukas*, see Woodroffe, *Garland of Letters*, 91.
7. In Patanjali's Yoga-Sutras (4:22) it is said that individual consciousness arises when purusha (Shiva), though immutable in its nature, is cast into buddhi, thus becoming its matrix. Vyasa's comment is that this consciousness is neither the same as nor different from buddhi. It is rather a prakritic copy, which is subject to change. These ideas will be clarified in the following chapters.
8. Woodroffe, *Garland of Letters*, 180.
9. "That which has been encoded with ideas in the inner microcosm, has been encoded with matter in the outer macrocosm" (S. Dasgupta, *The*

Study of Patañjali [Calcutta, 1920], 68). By this he means that the *paramanus*, which are the "atoms" of physical reality, are endowed with qualities corresponding to those of feelings and emotions. According to Hindu doctrines, there is no exception to the correspondence between mental modifications and their objective counterparts. Thus even abstract thoughts and passions match with "forms," which are somehow real, objective, and capable of being perceived.

10. On the psychological plane, this function of manas can be related to attentiveness. In the abovementioned Upanishadic text it is written: "I was elsewhere with manas, but I did not see or hear."

11. Kaushitaki-Upanishad 3:8.

12. Maitri-Upanishad 3:2, already quoted in Chapter III of this book.

13. In ancient Egyptian tradition the "subtle body" corresponds to the *skhem*, a term that may be translated as "power" (shakti), "forms," and even "vital force" (see W. Budge, *Gods of the Egyptians*, 163–64). There are also interesting correspondences with the doctrines related by Agrippa. He talked about "a celestial and aerial body, which some call the celestial vehicle of the soul, others the chariot of the soul. Through this middle thing . . . it is first infused into the middle point of the heart, which is the center of man's body [same view as that of Hinduism]" *(De occulta philosophia* 3:37). Agrippa goes on to say: "I call the sensitiveness of the soul [*eidolon*], that vivifying and rectifying power of the body, the origin of the senses; the soul itself manifests in this body its sensitive powers, perceives corporeal things by the body, governs it in this place, and nourishes itself in a body. In this sensitiveness [*eidolon*] two most principal powers predominate: namely, one that is called fantasy, or the imaginative or cogitative faculty, the other, which is called the sense of nature. . . . Man therefore by the nature of his body is under fate; the soul of man, by the sensitiveness of the soul, moves nature and fate, but by the mind is above fate" *(De occulta philosophia* 3:43).

14. Kaushitaki-Upanishad 3:2.

15. Maitri-Upanishad 2:6.

16. This corresponds to Agrippa's doctrine of the so-called "multiform *daimon*," or governing principle *(De occulta philosophia* 3:22). Agrippa speaks of a "sacred *daimon*" that "does not come from the 'stars' but from a higher cause, from the eternal Lord of the spirits." This principle has a universal character and dominates nature (samsara). Agrippa identifies this principle with the mind, the transcendent part of man, which "cannot be damned." After abandoning to their destiny (karma) the forces with which it is usually associated, the mind returns whole to its origin (3:36). Likewise, in Hindu doctrines, atman is not affected by good or evil deeds. Agrippa also mentions a second *daimon*, which is generated. According to some, this *daimon* is chosen by the soul prior to its descent in the body, and is influenced by the stars: it is "the principle that animates and preserves life, with which it animates the body."

17. Tantrattva 1:25.

Endnotes

CHAPTER V

1. Woodroffe, *Shakti and Shakta*, 409.
2. Kularnava-Tantra 2:7-8. Mahanirvana-Tantra 4:43–45.
3. Mahanirvana-Tantra 14:180. Further glorification of the kaulas is found in verses 183–93 of the same chapter. See also *Shakti and Shakta*, 141, 490–98.
4. In the Kalivilasa-Tantra (6:1–12) the pashus, viras, and divyas are related to the four ages of the present *mahayuga*. The divya's nature (*bhava*) informs the first two ages ("golden" and "silver" ages—Satya and Treta Yugas); the vira's nature informs the second and third ages ("silver" and "bronze"—Treta and Dvapara Yugas); the pashu's nature informs the last age (the "iron" age—Kali Yuga). Thus viras and divyas today represent the survivors of an extinguished spiritual race. According to the Jnana-Tantra "today there is hardly any nature [*bhava*] higher than a pashu's." This text either forbids the ritual with the *panchatattvas* or it requires it to be kept secret and revealed only to those who prove themselves to be viras and divyas.
5. We may recall the Tibetan tale of Naropa, who is looking for his teacher Tilopa. He keeps encountering him without being able to recognize him. For instance, Naropa comes across a man who asks him to help him finish off a woman he has just attacked. Naropa instead jumps on the man and frees the woman. Naropa suddenly finds himself alone, after what turns out to be a vision disappears. It was only a test; he then hears the voice of his teacher saying with a tone of irony in his voice: "I was that man." The same situation keeps occurring in other encounters, in which Tilopa is not recognized because he takes the disguise of a person performing or suggesting blameful acts.
6. Woodroffe, *Shakti and Shakta*, 153.
7. Manavadharmashastra XI:246, 261, 263.
8. "Verily this soul [atman] wanders here on earth from body to body, unovercome, as it seems, by the bright or the dark fruits of action" (Maitri-Upanishad 2:7).
9. Mahanirvana-Tantra 14:110.
10. Vairagya-Shakta 6:4.
11. Julius Evola, *The Doctrine of the Awakening*, trans. E. Mutton (London: Luzac, 1951), 107–10.
12. Indrabhuti, *Jnanasiddhi*. (Baroda: Bhattacharya, 1929), 29.
13. Mahanirvana-Tantra 1:59, 67.
14. "A sharpened edge of a razor, hard to traverse, a difficult path is this!" (Katha-Upanishad 1:3, 14).
15. Passage from the Mahabharata quoted in Mircea Eliade, *Yoga: Immortality and Freedom* (New York: Pantheon Books, 1958), 152.
16. "Sacrifice" in the context of a nondualistic doctrine can only have the meaning of a general orientation toward transcendence, since the idea of a personal god to whom oblations are to be made constitutes a reference

point only to those who are not enlightened (*mudhas*) and victim of their own ignorance. Various Tantric texts recall the words of the Bhagavad-Gita: "Who in all his work sees God, he is in truth unto God: God is his worship, God is his offering, offered by God in the fire of God" (4:24).

17. "The world is in the bonds of action, unless the action is consecration. Let thy actions then be pure, free from the bonds of desire" (3:29). Also: "He has attained liberation: he is free from all bonds, his mind has found peace in wisdom, and his work is a holy sacrifice. The work of such a man is pure" 4:23.

18. Bhagavad-Gita 11, passim.

19. Von Glasenapp, *Buddhistiche Mysterien*, 30.

20. W. Y. Evans-Wentz, *Tibetan Yoga and Secret Doctrines* (London: Oxford University Press, 1958), 138.

21. Hatha-Yoga-Pradipika 3:1.

22. Woodroffe, *Shakti and Shakta*, 643–45.

CHAPTER VI

1. *De occulta philosophia* 3:3.

2. Giuseppe Tucci, *Teoria e pratica dei mandala* (Rome, 1949), 51.

3. Kaushitaki-Upanishad 2:2. Dasgupta, *The Study of Patañjali* (Calcutta, 1920), 149–50.

4. Western initiatory traditions talk about a "univocal generation," in which "the son is the same as the father in every aspect. This generation is the power of the word, which is formed by the mind [*mens*]" (Agrippa, *De occulta philosophia* 3:36).

5. Mahanirvana-Tantra 8:264–65.

6. Alexandra David-Neel, in her *Mystics and Magicians of Tibet* (1932), related this episode: The Dalai Lama, surprised by her knowledge of Tibetan doctrines, asked her who had been her teacher. He was utterly surprised to learn from her that one of the Tibetan texts expounding those doctrines had long since been translated into French, and that many people had learned about them. He then went on to say, "If some foreigners have learned our language and read our sacred texts, they must have missed their deeper meaning." The same applies to the majority of orientalists.

7. Alexandra David-Neel explained that the Tibetan word for "to imagine" is *migspa*. *Migspa* consists in concentrating until the subjective thought being imagined materializes. *Migspa* is an active trance in which events and places that are being imagined completely replace those that are perceived in the ordinary state of wakefulness.

8. A similar technique is the Buddhist technique of the so-called *kasina*. See Evola, *Doctrine of the Awakening*, 206–28.

9. Evans-Wentz, *Tibetan Yoga*, 301.

Endnotes

10. See Eliade's bibliography in his *Yoga: Immortality and Freedom*, 370–72; also, chapter 2, "Techniques for Autonomy," 47–100.
11. See the texts quoted in Evans-Wentz, *Tibetan Yoga*, 128–30, 138.
12. The most sophisticated system of de-identification techniques is found in the canonical texts of early Buddhism. See my *Doctrine of the Awakening*, 134–148.
13. Evans-Wentz, *Tibetan Yoga*, 128–29.
14. The Hatha-Yoga-Pradipika (4:66-67; 84-88) contains indications on how to use sounds in order to neutralize the mental organ. The goal pursued here is the achievement of the last two phases of samadhi, and suspension of breath seems to be associated with practice. In the region of the heart some sounds are manifested. The inner sound (*nada*) at first is strong and resembles various things, such as a bell, waves, thunder, or rain. The mind must keep concentrating on these subtle sounds, excluding all other perceptions, until it becomes fixed and until it has successfully removed the limitation that it represents for the I. "Just like a hunter, the sound first attracts, ties, and finally slays the mind. . . . When the inner organ, similar to a deer, pauses and listens to a sound, a skilled hunter is able to kill it" (4:92, 94, 99).
15. In Eliade's *Yoga*, 72–73, we find an interesting description of "the subject of fire as it is taught today (the meditation begins with concentration, *dharana*, on some glowing coals placed before the yogin). Not only does it reveal to the yogin the phenomenon of combustion and its deeper meaning; it allows him, in addition: (1) to identify the physicochemical process taking place in the coal with the process of combustion that occurs in the human body; (2) to identify the fire before him with the fire of the sun, etc.; (3) to unify the several contents of all these fires, in order to obtain a vision of existence as 'fire'; (4) to penetrate within this cosmic process, now on the astral plane (the sun), now on the physiological plane (the human body), and finally even on the plane of infinitesimals ("the seeds of fire"); (5) to "master" the inner fire, by virtue of *pranayama*, suspension of respiration (respiration = vital fire); (6) finally, through a new "penetration," to extend this "mastery" to the glowing coals before him (for, if the process of combustion is exactly the same from one limit of the universe to the other, any partial mastery of the phenomenon infallibly leads to its "mastery" *in toto*)."
16. Concerning the variety of the psychic and extrasensory experiences, see Rama Prasad, *Nature's Inner Forces*, 161–74. There is also a famous saying in the *Corpus hermeticum*: "Having been strengthened by God, I contemplate not through the eyes but through the intellectual energy of the sensory powers."
17. Svetasvatara-Upanishad 3:18–19: "Though in a nine-gated city [the human body] embodied, back and forth to the external hovers the soul, the controller of the whole world, both the stationary and the moving. Without foot or hand, he is swift and a seizer! He sees without eye; he hears without ear!"

18. The general meaning of this exercise is found in this passage of Agrippa (*De occulta philosophia*): "The air [*prana*] is the body of our sensitive spirit's life; it does not correspond to any sensible object, but it has a high spiritual value. Nevertheless, the sensitive soul must vivify the air by which it is engulfed. It must also experience the objects that act on it, surrounded by a *vivified air that is attached to the spirit, which we call the 'living air'*" (italics mine).

19. "So just as those who do not know the spot might go over a hidden treasure of gold again and again, but do not find it, even so all creatures here go day by day to that Brahma world (*brahma-loka*) [in deep sleep], but do not find it; for truly they are carried away by what is false" (Chandogya-Upanishad 8:3, 2).

20. "Assuredly, this is the heat of Brahma, the supreme, the immortal, the bodiless—even the warmth of the body. . . . Now, although it [i.e., the heat] is manifest, verily it is hidden in the ether [of the heart]. . . . The ether storehouse of the heart is bliss, is the supreme abode! This is ourself, our yoga too; and this, the heat of fire and sun" (Maitri-Upanishad 6:27). In this, as well as in other cases, it is difficult to separate in the texts what is typical of a preliminary practice from what is achieved in a higher realization, which is obtained by persevering in the same direction.

21. Hatha-Yoga-Pradipika 2:49: "He should do *kumbhaka* until he feels that the whole body from head to toe is suffused by prana; then he should slowly exhale through the left nostril."

22. It is said that this shift may occur easily if one proceeds gradually, by concentrating first on an immaterial spot in the middle of the head, then on a spot located around the larynx, and finally on the heart.

23. See Evans-Wentz, *Tibetan Yoga*, chapter 3, pp. 226–29.

24. "Now the soul (*atman*) is the bridge [dam], the separation for keeping these worlds apart. Over that bridge [or dam] crosses neither day, nor night, nor old age, nor death, nor sorrow, nor well-doing, nor evil-doing. . . . Therefore, verily, upon crossing that bridge, if one is blind, he becomes no longer blind; if he is sick, he becomes no longer sick. Therefore, verily, upon crossing that bridge, the night appears even as day, for that Brahma world is ever illumined" (Chandogya-Upanishad 8:4:1–2). Also: "When there is no darkness, then there is no day or night" (Svetasvatara-Upanishad 4:18).

25. Evans-Wentz, *Tibetan Yoga*, 225–26.

26. It is possible to find a correspondence with the mudras in the Western magical tradition. Agrippa, for instance, talks about representations of "sacred numbers" through particular gestures, which indicate "names with inexpressible qualities, which one should not pronounce aloud."

27. In the context of hatha yoga, the yogin comes to exercise control over muscles that usually do not depend on his will. He also becomes capable of controlling the excreting organs. Such a control is also exhibited in the course of Tantric sexual practices by men, in relation to the capability of reabsorbing the semen spilled during intercourse, and by women in

relation to the capability of contracting the vaginal muscles around the male organ until they totally immobilize it.

28. It is said that yogins can transmit their magical immobility to their clothes. At the peak of the yogin's meditation, his clothes become stiff and do not move even when a strong wind is blowing, as if they were protected or permeated by a magical aura.

29. It is said that the cross-legged position of the two main asanas has the purpose of isolating the body from earthly undercurrents. This isolation is strengthened if the yogin sits on a special herb or if he sits on a tiger's or antelope's skin. The influence of earthly undercurrents and the closing of the circuit, which is effected by asanas and by mudras, can only be perceived by those yogins who have developed a high degree of subtle sensibility. Whether perceived or not, however, the effects of these negative forces are supposed to be an objective reality.

CHAPTER VII

1. "Throwing away one's clothes" is a symbol employed in ancient Western initiatory practices. In a Nassen text, a mention is made of the spiritual man who throws away his clothes and becomes the groom, having received true virility from the Virgin, and being clothed only with his power. A central theme in Alexandrian Gnosticism was that of the Perfect Man, who descends into the Virgin's womb, removes the impurity contaminating the "firstborn of water" (to be associated with Shakti's descending current), washes himself, and drinks from the living waters. By doing this he burns his "savage form" and transforms it into a "dress of power."

2. There is a parallel allegory in the legendary life of Tilopa, who was one of the great teachers of the Tibetan Tantric "Direct Path." After a journey filled with many ordeals (which symbolize the process of purification) he finally encounters Dakini, the primordial Woman, or a Shakti of divine beauty, who is sitting on a throne. He strips her naked by tearing her clothes off and then rapes her on her throne.

3. This can be compared with Tilopa's symbolic journey. In medieval chivalric literature we find analogous themes in a cryptic form: the journeys, trials, and adventures that the knights undergo in the name of a "Woman."

4. Woodroffe, *Shakti and Shakta*, 529; Mahanirvana-Tantra 1:53.

5. Shrichakrasmbhara-Tantra, 61.

6. It seems that Goethe claimed this privilege for himself.

7. Panchakrama 6:30. Also quoted in von Glasenapp, *Buddhistische Mysterien*, 174.

8. Prapanchasara-Tantra (23:56–58): "Under no circumstance may one disobey a guru. The disciple must immediately do as ordered, without hesitations and without trying to determine whether the order is right or wrong."

9. Evans-Wentz, *Tibetan Yoga*, chapter 5.

10. This level is characterized by the release from all bonds, from natural

impulses, and from samskaras; by inner neutrality *(upeksha);* and by the revelation of the reality hidden behind various powers.

Chapter VIII

1. There is an analogy between the Shaktic experience and the ancient Roman concept of *numen,* which was a god conceived essentially under the species of a power *(shakti).*

2. In the Shrichakrasambhara-Tantra it is written: "Every visible object should be considered a divine being whose real nature is *shunyata."* In the Tantraraja the various phases of the contemplation of Shakti are related to various parts of a graphic symbol, the so-called shri-yantra. The following are the phases of this contemplation: (1) all material things, the senses, the mind, are shakti; (2) All these particular shaktis are but various parts of one primordial power *(adya-shakti);* (3) the apprentice himself, both in his essential principle *(atma)* and in his mind and body, forms one thing with the supreme Shakti. This is expressly stated in the Mahanirvana-Tantra (1:16): "Thou, O Devi, art my very self. There is no difference between me and thee."

3. On this, see Woodroffe, *Shakti and Shakta,* 420. There is a strong formal analogy between this rite and the Roman Catholic Mass, which is supposed to induce the "real presence" of Christ under the eucharistic species.

4. B. de Rachelwiltz, *Egitto magico e religioso* (Turin, 1961), 140.

5. See Evans-Wentz, *Tibetan Yoga,* 173–76.

6. Gandharva-Tantra 21:2.

7. Mahanirvana-tantra 3:43.

8. Woodroffe, *Shakti and Shakta,* 105–24. Tantrism practices the so-called *matrika-nyasa,* which is the *nyasa* of the "letters" and of the "little mothers," and which has an inner dimension *(antarmatrika-nyasa)* and a ritual dimension *(bahyamatrika-nyasa).* This *nyasa* consists in mentally positioning the letters of the Sanskrit alphabet inside the six chakras (subtle centers) and in various parts of the body, putting one's hand over them, and pronouncing the corresponding letters.

9. *De occulta philosophia* 3:13.

10. An analogous practice, called *shambhavi-mudra,* is described in the Hatha-Yoga-Pradipika (4:36–37): "Fixing the mind inwardly and fixing the eyes without blinking on an external object. . . . It is rightfully called *shambhavi-mudra,* when mind and prana are absorbed by the object, when the eyes become rigid in the contemplation of the object."

11. Mahanirvana-Tantra 5:105.

12. *De occulta philosophia* 1:33.

13. Mahanirvana-Tantra 3:31.

14. Arthur Avalon [Sir John Woodroffe], *The Serpent Power,* 7th ed. (Madras: Ganesh, 1964), 169.

15. "Every voice, therefore, that is significative, first of all signifies by the influence of the celestial harmony; secondly, by the imposition of man, although oftentimes otherwise by this than by that. But when both significations meet in any voice or name, which are put upon them by the said harmony or men, then that name is with a double virtue, viz., natural and arbitrary, made most efficacious to act, as often as it shall be uttered in due place and time, and seriously, with an intention exercised upon the matter rightly disposed, and that can naturally be acted upon by it" Agrippa, *De philosophia occulta* (1:70).

Chapter IX

1. Mahanirvana-Tantra 5:24. It is also said that if a ritual is performed without *panchatattva*, "that siddhi which is the object of sadhana is never attained thereby, and obstacles are encountered at every step" (Ibid., 5:13).

2. Ibid., 7:103–11. *Mudra* was originally the name of a plant or of a seed with aphrodisiac characteristics. Subsequently the term came to designate the vira's partner.

3. This was the meaning of the ancient Roman ritual of the *lectisternium*. We may also recall the institution, in pagan Rome, of the *tresviri epulones* and, later on, of the *septemviri epulones*, which were a priestly body presiding at sacred banquets.

4. Woodroffe, *Shakti and Shakta*, 95–105.

5. Brihad-Aranyaka-Upanishad 6:4:19–22.

6. Mahanirvana-Tantra 5:24.

7. Alexandra David-Neel recounted Tibetan practices aimed at prolonging the man's life through sexual union by repeatedly provoking the woman's orgasm and withholding ejaculation.

8. Rig-Veda (10:85): "When one drinks the juice of the plant, he should imagine to be drinking soma. However, nobody knows the Brahmans' soma. It is kept secret by them."

9. In Homer's *Hymn to Demeter* (480–83 A.D.) it is written: "Those who have not known sacred orgies and those who have participated in them do not share the same fate after death."

10. Mahanirvana-Tantra 11:108.

11. Ibid., 6:196.

12. One myth, concerning the divine man Kasha, who was set on fire by the Asuras (= the Titans), parallels the main theme of Orphic-Dionysian practices. According to Orphism, the Titans were stricken by a heavenly thunder for having killed and devoured Dionysius Zagreus. Humans are believed to have been created from their ashes; thus they are a mixture of Dionysian and Titanic elements.

13. Mahanirvana-Tantra 10:112.

14. Ibid., 8:207.

15. Woodroffe, *Shakti and Shakta*, 583.

16. The women that are recommended for the ritual are not women but teenagers. However, one should consider the rapid physical and sexual development of Hindu women. Unless one finds a younger girl, the maximum age is twenty. Women who are older than twenty "do not have any occult power." In China, Taoist sexual practices recommended the use of teenagers as well.

17. M. Eliade wrote, concerning the magical-ritual nudity of the *yogini* (the vira's partner): "If, in the presence of the naked woman, one does not find in one's inmost being the same terrifying emotion that one feels before the revelation of the cosmic mystery, there is no rite, there is only a secular act, with all the familiar consequences (strengthening of the karmic chain, etc.)" (*Yoga: Immortality and Freedom*, 259).

18. In some Tantric literature woman is depicted as a tiger stealing man's vital principle and eating it.

19. Hatha-Yoga-Pradipika 3:42–43.

20. Ibid., 3:85.

21. The biblical text subject to this esoteric interpretation is Numbers 25:6–8.

22. Julius Evola, *Metaphysics of Sex*, (Rochester, Vt: Inner Traditions, 1989), chapter 3.

23. M. Eliade, *Yoga: Immortality and Freedom*, 255.

24. Mahanirvana-Tantra 7:111.

25. Woodroffe, *Shakti and Shakta*, 649.

CHAPTER X

1. Woodroffe, *Shakti and Shakta*, 277. Also: "Whatever is here, that is there. What is there, that again is here. He obtains death after death, who seems to see a difference here." (Katha-Upanishad 4:10).

2. Shivagama, 14.

3. One Upanishad explicitly states that when all the mental processes are neutralized, the state that ensues is "different from deep sleep." In the Hatha-Yoga-Pradipika it is said that the state of samadhi is experienced by one who maintains a clear mind while remaining in a waking state resembling sleep.

4. For a more detailed critique of Jung's theories, see the essay found in J. G. Gichtel, *Introduzione alla magia* 3:411ff.

5. Julius Evola, *Eros and the Mysteries of Love*, 49–54.

6. According to the Yoga-Kundali-Upanishad, one of the greatest obstacles is eliminated by allowing the semen to flow upward.

7. In a Hermetic symbol are two birds, one with wings, the other without wings. The former strives to drag the latter along; the latter wishes to remain on the ground. Hermetic arts attempt to reconcile these two birds, which represent opposing tendencies in human beings.

Endnotes

8. Arthur Avalon, *The Serpent Power*, 131.
9. Evans-Wentz, *Tibetan Yoga*, 190.
10. Hatha-Yoga-Pradipika (3:109) mentions a widow who sits by two rivers (symbols of pingala and ida). She must be forcibly stripped and raped, "for she leads to the supreme seat of Vishnu." The widow is kundalini, or Shakti without her mate. The clothes she wears are particular forms behind which she hides. We may also consider the esoteric interpretation of a Hellenistic myth in which Zeus chases his own mother, Rhea (her name means "flowing" = Shakti): "When Rhea took the form of a serpent *[kundalini]*, Zeus assumed that form too, and after tying her with 'Heracles' noose,' he possessed her. The symbol of this transformation is Hermes' scepter." This symbol represents the image of the three main subtle currents within the human being, which are considered in hatha yoga.
11. As in Evola's original Italian, only nine syllables are given here.
12. In the gesture that dispenses favors *(vara-mudra)* the hand is held horizontally with the palm facing upward; the fingers are kept close together, and the thumb is folded across the hand, touching the base of the ring finger. In the other gesture the hand is raised, palm facing the observer, while the fingers are in the same position.
13. In the symbolic popular iconography, Sadashiva is represented as having five faces and ten hands, which hold as many objects. These objects, such as a trident, a spear, a sacrificial sword, a thunderbolt, the great snake Dahana, a lamp, a sting, and a noose, represent various divine attributes.
14. *Itara* has been variously interpreted in regard to its power of transcending *kala* (temporality); *itara-linga* is an allegory of Shiva's virility in this particular, timeless aspect.
15. Avalon, *The Serpent Power*, 95.
16. The figure of the eternal guru could be compared with the Kabbalist Adam Kadmon, a "gigantic, ineffable man" whose substance is pure light; some schools of Alexandrian Gnosticism have talked about this figure.
17. The reader will find a detailed discussion of the Hermetic-alchemical equivalent to the passage through the "Seven" in my *La tradizione ermetica*. The esoteric doctrine of the chakras is also partially found in the writings of a Christian mystic, J. G. Gichtel (*Introduzione alla magia* 2:16ff). As far as the septenary correspondences in reference to planets, heavenly hierarchies and bodily organs are concerned, see Agrippa, *De occulta philosophia* 2:70, 1:22ff.
18. The correspondences between the two opposite snakes and pingala and ida have been emphasized by B. de Rachewiltz in his *Egitto magico e religioso* (Turin, 1961).
19. There is a Western correspondence to the Tantric teaching concerning the *muladhara-chakra*, which is a center from which kundalini begins a process of regeneration. This correspondence is found in the writings of Agrippa. He mentions: "There is in man's body a certain little bone, which the Hebrews call *luz*, of the bigness of a pulse that is husked, which is subject to no corruption, neither is it overcome with fire, but it is always pre-

served unhurt, out of which, as they say, as a plant out of the seed, our animal bodies shall in the resurrection of the dead spring up. And these virtues are not cleared by the reason, but by experience." (*De occulta phil.* 1:20). A. Reghini, in his introduction to the Italian translation of Agrippa's *De occulta philosophia*, concluded that *luz*, in Aramaic, is the name of the coccyx, a cone-shaped bone at the base of the spinal cord. *Luz* was also the ancient name of the city that Jacob called Bethel ("The House of the Lord") after he fell asleep on a stone and after he had a vision; this terrifying vision was that of the dwelling place of the Lord, on which Jacob was lying (Genesis 28:11–19). Reghini also mentioned some traditions according to which, in the proximity of Luz-Bethel, there is a "hidden gateway leading to a path that runs through the city" (a symbol of the states that correspond to the various chakras).

Chapter XI

1. Yoga-Sutras 2:49.
2. Retention of breath can be used, for instance, in some practices of black magic, called *phowa*, in order to enter other people's bodies. Breath retention is also employed by Hindu fakirs (ascetics) in order to facilitate hibernation, or the suspension of the body's vital functions for a certain amount of time, in which the body may even be buried.
3. "When breath is suspended then discursive thinking is also suspended. He who has power over his mind can also control prana" (Hatha-Yoga-Pradipika 4:21).
4. Maitri-Upanishad 6:34.
5. Svetasvatara-Upanishad 2:8.
6. The "destruction of the I" (*niratma-katvam*) is related to "breaking the limit of breath retention" and to "becoming one with what is without limitations, once prana runs through sushumna."
7. Evola, *The Doctrine of the Awakening*, 182–205. In these pages I discuss the dhyanas of early Buddhism. The last dhyana seems to correspond to the suspension of breath practiced in yoga.
8. Franz M. Cumont, *The Mysteries of Mithras*, trans. T. J. McCormack (New York: Dover, 1956), 135.
9. Evans-Wentz, *Tibetan Yoga*, 173–75.
10. Ibid., 178.
11. Swedenborg, the Nordic mystic and visionary, used to talk about an inner breathing that took place when external breathing was completely suspended. This suspension used to take place unconsciously, even during sleep. When that happened, he entered a kind of trance in which he could see and communicate with angels and spirits.
12. The state in which breathing is suspended, the body is absolutely still, and the flux of mental formations is interrupted.
13. Svetasvatara-Upanishad 2:13; Hatha-Yoga-Pradipika 2:77.

14. Evans-Wentz, *Tibetan Yoga*, 195. Also: "Fog, smoke, sun, fire, wind, fire-flies, lighting a crystal, a moon. These are the preliminary appearances that produce the manifestation of Brahma in yoga" (Svetasvetara-Upanishad 2:11).

15. The natural habitat of Tibet, characterized by glaciers, high mountains, and vast plateaus, seems to be one of the reasons why yogic traditions were preserved more faithfully there than in other places. The Chandogya-Upanishad (8:15) and the Maitri-Upanishad (6:30) exhort the apprentice to choose a "clean place" and a "pure place."

16. Hatha-Yoga-Pradipika 1:11.

17. In some texts—including the Hatha-Yoga-Pradipika itself—the reader may come to the conclusion that the descriptions therein contained are mainly of physiological processes. This could generate a misunderstanding, since in true yoga there is no such thing as purely physiological practices.

18. "If one fixes a strong lock on the entrance door of breath; if in that terrible darkness one makes the spirit a lamp; if the jewel of the *jina* [conqueror] touches the supreme heaven above, Kahna says, one accomplishes *nirvana* while still enjoying existence" (Eliade, *Yoga*, 268).

19. According to the Shiva-Samhita (3:29–41), the first phase of pranayama is characterized by the decrease of feces, urine, and sleep. In the second phase perspiration occurs. In the third phase the body begins to shiver, to jump, and eventually to levitate.

20. In Tibet one of the magical powers obtained by the yogin consists in being able to cover great distances without feeling tired, running at a very fast pace, and almost in a trancelike state.

21. In Zen Buddhism one of the trials that the disciple has to face consists in submitting himself to strangulation at the hands of a teacher.

22. A. Avalon described the experience of kundalini's awakening. The Westerner who experienced it recalled feeling at the mercy of a greater power: "I felt frightened, as the Power seemed something which could consume me" (*The Serpent Power*, 21).

23. "Courage is required. One should expect to find his path barred by all kinds of forces. A bandit or an anarchist can easily reach God, because they know no fears. They only need to be shown the right direction" (Siravanda Sarasvati, *La pratique de la meditation* [Paris, 1950], 398).

24. Evans-Wentz, *Tibetan Yoga*, 192–93.

25. Ibid., 204–6.

26. Ibid., 201.

27. Cumont, *Mysteries of Mithra*, 38, 137.

28. Evans-Wentz, *Tibetan Yoga*, 132–33.

CHAPTER XII

1. Hatha-Yoga-Pradipika 4:17.

2. These spheres exemplify states of "nonidentity" and correspond to seven

planets and to seven doors. In Hindu metaphysics they are states in which *maya-shakti's* law of dualism is fully operative.

3. Franz M. Cumont, *The Mysteries of Mithras,* trans. T. J. McCormack (New York: Dover, 1956). See also *Corpus hermeticum* 1:26.

4. Kularvana-Tantra 9:9.

5. G. G. Scholem, *Major Trends in Jewish Mysticism* (New York: Schocken Books, 1946), 62ff.

6. S. Dasgupta, *Obscure Religious Cults* (Calcutta: K. L. Mukhopadhyay, 1969), 292ff.

7. W. Budge, *God of the Egyptians,* 163–64.

8. *De occulta philosophia* 3:44.

9. Magnien, *Les mystères d'Eleusis* (Paris: Payot, 1938), 61–62.

10. Mahanirvana-Tantra 14:126.

11. "The fact that yogin does not display his powers in public is explainable by the preliminary condition for their achievement, namely, by the yogin's absolute indifference for the things of this world" (Rossel, *Die psychologischen Grundlagen der Yogapraxis* [Stuttgrat, 1928], 85).

12. *The Yoga-Sutra of Patañjali,* trans. G. Feuerstein (Rochester, Vt.: Inner Traditions, 1991).

13. Evans-Wentz, *Tibetan Yoga,* 198–200.

14. In the Hatha-Yoga-Pradipika (4:106) it is said that the yogin is "free from remembering and from forgetting."

15. Woodroffe, *Shakti and Shakta,* 648.

16. Evans-Wentz, *Tibet's Great Yogi Milarepa* (London, 1934), 35.

17. Woodroffe, *Shakti and Shakta,* 649. The *chakravarti's* function is to serve as a "hub" or "axis." Literally the term means "wheel spinner," a being who does not take part in its motion. In this case the adept partakes of this function.

CONCLUSION

1. Nirvana came to be seen mainly as a refuge from this "sorrowful world." I am not pleased to report that in no work other than my *Doctrine of the Awakening* it is possible to have an idea of what early Buddhism stood for, prior to its ensuing decadence.

2. René Guenon, *Man and His Becoming According to Vedanta.*

3. What I have just said will probably disappoint those who know only the minimalist, modified, and practical yoga that has been imported into the West, as well as those frivolous people who believe that through this or that exercise it is possible to achieve goodness knows what.

4. Julius Evola, *L'arco e la clava* (Milan, 1967), chapter 15.

5. I quote the meaningful words of a Tantric author: "Both Sankara's *jnana-yoga* and Ramanuja's *bhakti-yoga* share a pessimistic perspective. Conversely, in the *Tantras* one does not find reference to 'valley of tears,' or

to 'house of torments,' and to similar designations with which transcendalist *darshanas* express their contempt for the world. . . . Those who practice Tantrism achieve liberation while enjoying the goods of the world which the followers of other schools deprive themselves of." (Woodroffe, *Tantrattva* 2:34).

6. A typical example of the vulgarization of Tantrism for the use of Western-ers is a book by O. Garrison, *Tantra: The Yoga of Sex* (New York, 1964). Unfortunately, this book has also been translated into Italian. This book deserves no rating, since it is filled with blunders and inspired by a dull spiritualism. The author, an American, says that he was inspired by a guru "who runs a successful legal office in Bombay."(!!!) Another ex-ample of the poor quality of adaptations of Tantrism to Western stan-dards is represented by the "Tantric Order of America," which used to publish a journal in which the readers were reminded that "there is no amount of money large enough to reward a tantric initiation." At least in this "order" there was no pretension of spiritualism, since there were many scandals and lawsuits against its members. These "tantrikas," espe-cially their Great Master, who took the modest name of "Om the Omnipo-tent," seduced quite a few beautiful American girls; the lawsuits were brought against them, not so much because the girls complained about the "initiations" they underwent, but because their parents were not so thrilled about the whole thing (in those days there was not yet the "beat generation").

7. These ideas should always be within the context of a general worldview and of ethics, leaving aside anything related to initiation and yoga.

APPENDIX ONE

1. See W. Y. Evans-Wentz, *The Tibetan Book of the Dead* (London: Oxford University Press, 1927); and by the same author, *Tibetan Yoga and Secret Doctrines* (London: Oxford University Press, 1935).

2. Evans-Wentz, *Tibetan Book of the Dead*, 213.

3. In texts such as the Kaushitaki-Upanishad, the Moon, which is considered the symbolic place where those who are carried along the *pitriyana* are dissolved and "sacrificed to the gods," was also considered a potential transit area on the "way of the gods." This area was once and for all left behind by those who knew the answers to given questions. If one is not up to it, one's destiny takes place "according to his deeds (karma)." One of the answers is "I am the truth." This answer, according to a conven-tional interpretation, means "whatever is other than the sense organs *(deva)* and the vital breaths (prana)."

4. Evans-Wentz, *Tibetan Book of the Dead*, xxvii.

5. This book has been translated into English by F. M. Comper with the title *The Book of the Craft of Dying* (London, 1917).

6. *In Platonis Phaedro*, 14.

7. This ephemeral I is a pale reflection of an eternal form, which is its

"name," and which preexists it on a supratemporal plane. At death the reflection is reabsorbed, the same way during sleep the normal waking consciousness is reabsorbed and "disappears." Only he who has become "a living being," who has achieved the awakening, will assume at death that form and realize its name. His name is inscribed in the "Book of the Eternal," or in the "Tree of Life," to use an Egyptian expression.

8. More specifically, it is possible for the life flux to fall back into the subhuman kingdoms; this is the true meaning, (as the late Lama Dawa-Samdup remarked (Evans-Wentz, *Tibetan Book of the Dead*, 44), of the teaching, expressed in a popular and symbolic form, concerning "animal rebirths."

9. According to the ancient Hellenistic mysteries' teachings, this is how the *nous*, or mind, becomes separated from the *psyche*, or soul. The form that is taken by the former is the *soma pneumatikon*, the "body of pneuma," or "spiritual body," which participates of the nature of air and of luminous ether; by joining the superior principle, it survives death.

10. Evans-Wentz, *Tibetan Yoga*, 80.

11. Evans-Wentz, *Tibetan Book of the Dead*, 94–95.

12. Ibid., 151.

13. Ibid., 91.

14. Evans-Wentz, *Tibetan Yoga*, 233.

15. Brihad-Aranyaka-Upanishad 4:3:38, 4:4:1–4.

16. René Guenon, *L'erreur spirite* (Paris, 1923).

17. Evans-Wentz, *Tibetan Book of the Dead*, 104.

18. Ibid., 103. Agrippa (*De occulta phil.* 3:41) claimed that afterlife experiences are not real events, but only "mirages apprehended by the imagination. . . . Orpheus called them 'people of dreams.' There is also a saying: The gates of Pluto cannot be unlocked; within is a people of dreams."

19. Even the beliefs that one had while alive, concerning the afterlife, may play a role in the "cosmic dream" of the deceased.

20. Evans-Wentz, *Tibetan Book of the Dead*, 131.

21. Ibid.

22. Ibid., 132. The text suggests that if one does not succeed in remembering the teachings laid out in the Bardo Thödol by keeping the mind focused on one thought and by remaining aware, "one's hearing of religious lore—although it be like an ocean in its vastness—is of no avail."

23. Evans-Wentz, *Tibetan Yoga*, 240.

24. This can only happen through a vigorous spiritual action or on the basis of various propensities that were acquired or nourished by practicing the cult of unrestrained and destructive Dionysian deities.

25. Evans-Wentz, *Tibetan Book of the Dead*, 156.

26. Ibid., 176.

27. Ibid., 177.

28. Evans-Wentz, *Tibetan Yoga*, 245.

29. Evans-Wentz, *Tibetan Book of the Dead*, 166–67.
30. Ibid., 180.
31. Ibid., 178.
32. Ibid., 188.
33. Ibid., 191.
34. Evans-Wentz, *Tibetan Yoga*, 18.

APPENDIX TWO

1. Julius Evola, *Eros and the Mysteries of Love*, (Rochester, Vt.: Inner Traditions, 1983).
2. Dante Alighieri, *The New Life*, trans. Thomas Okey (London: Dent, 1906).
3. Ibid., 3:24-31 (italics mine).
4. This is also the case of the French term *salut* and of the German term *heil*. According to the symbolism of the Minnesingers (who were the German equivalent of the Worshipers of Love), *heil* (well-being) is considered to be the "woman's" (Vrore Saelde's) "son."
5. Dante, *The New Life*, 19:49–52.
6. Ibid., 2:13–17 (italics mine).

INDEX

Index

De-identification. *See* Samyama

Death, process of, 196–201; devayana (path), 192; identification with devas during, 195, 198–201; pitriyana (path), 192, 233. *See also* Bardo

Detachment. *See* Mukti

Devatas (deities): evocation of, 102–5, 111–12; identification with, 101–6, 170–71, 195, 198–201; invocation of, 105–15

Devi (goddesses), 5, 20, 53, 55. *See also* Shakti

Dharana. *See* Samyama

Dharma (truth), 57–58, 59, 60, 97, 211; adharma, 58, 59. *See also* Karma

Dhyana. *See* Samyama

Divine couple. *See* Maithuna

Divya (divine), 55, 66, 68, 93, 138–39, 182–85, 189, 211

Ekagriya. *See* Manas

Elements. *See* Matter

Eliade, Mircea, 9, 91, 228, 231

Emptiness. *See* Mukti

Enlightenment. *See* Mukti; Samyama

Enoch, 179, 181

Entelechy, 49

Evans-Wentz, W.Y., 8–9, 65, 196, 202, 203, 204, 231

Evocation, 103–4, 102–5, 111–12, 113–15, 129

Evola, Julius, background of, ix–xv

Evolution. *See* Yugas

Fascism, xii

Fire, 223

Freud, Sigmund, 142, 202

Gandharva-Tantra, 105

Garrison, O., 233

Ghrina (disgust), 96

Guenon, René, xiv, 36–37, 186–87

Guhyas, 108

Gunas (powers of prakriti), 40–41, 47–48, 54, 211; rajas (activity), 40–41, 48, 54, 55; sattva (stability), 40, 48, 54, 55, 66; tamas (passivity), 40, 41, 47, 48, 54, 141

Guru (teacher), 74–75, 98–99, 225

Hallucinations, 174–75, 176, 198–201

Hamsah (vital principle), 160, 162, 211

Hermetica, xii

Ida. *See* Kundalini, paths of

Identification, 17, 83–86, 101–6, 170–71, 195, 198–201, 213, 228

Illusion. *See* Reality

Immortality, 180–82

Individuation, 41–47, 50–52. *See also* Samskaras

Indriyas (senses), 44–47, 82, 86, 223; tanmatras (supersenses), 44, 45–46, 150–57; transformation of, 107–8. *See also* Kaya

Intoxicants, 76–77, 116–17, 119, 120–23, 125–26

Invocation, 105–15

Ishmaelites, 99

Ishvara (lord), 39, 40, 58, 211

Jung, Carl, 142

Kali, 3, 4, 5, 7, 30–31, 61, 104, 135, 211

Kali Yuga (dark age), 2, 3–4, 15, 54, 188–89

Kankukas. *See* Maya-shakti

Karma, 42, 51, 57–58, 211, 216; and death, 191, 192, 200, 201–2; transcendence of, 60–61, 99–100, 222. *See also* Dharma

Kaula (initiate), 53–56, 59–60, 93–94, 211–12

Kaya (body): causal, 48, 141, 143, 155–56; correct use of, 66–68; material, 48–49, 141; nirmana-kaya (transformed), 177–85, 204; perception of, 86–90; subtle, 48, 49–52, 141, 143, 146–47, 220. *See also* Indriyas; Yoga

Knowledge; in democracy, 16; types of, 10–14, 17, 218

Krishna, 60–61, 100

Kula (kinship), 96–97

Kumbhaka. *See* Pranayama

Kundalini (latent energy), 144–45, 212, 229–30; awakening of, 138, 146–49, 159–69, 171–73, 231; and sex ritual, 145–46; Shakti as, 47, 144, 145; dangers of, 173–75; effects of, 167, 169–70, 172, 178; and liberation, 177–82. *See also* Chakras

Kundalini, paths of: ida, 147, 168–69, 171–73, 211; pingala, 147, 166, 168–69, 171–73, 213; sushumna, 148, 158, 168, 171–72, 178, 213

Lajja (shame), 95